Controversial Pain Syndromes of the Arm

Albrecht Wilhelm

Controversial Pain Syndromes of the Arm

Pathogenesis and Surgical Treatment of Resistant Cases

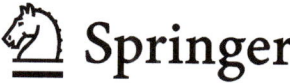 Springer

Albrecht Wilhelm
Aschaffenburg
Germany

ISBN 978-3-642-54512-2   ISBN 978-3-642-54513-9   (eBook)
DOI 10.1007/978-3-642-54513-9
Springer Heidelberg New York Dordrecht London

Library of Congress Control Number: 2014949162

Printed on acid-free paper

Springer is part of Springer Science+Business Media (www.springer.com)

This monography is dedicated to my dear wife Annemarie and to both of our children, Andrea and Wolfgang, with thanks for their understanding and for their support of my work.

Foreword

Albrecht Wilhelm is one of the General Surgeons who had training in the entire field of surgery. His career started where it should start for a surgeon, in the anatomy lab. There he learned the meticulous dissection technique when he dissected the neural innervations of the joints of the upper extremity. From this knowledge he later developed a standardized technique for the operative denervation of the wrist.

From very early on hand surgery was hobby and field of special interest of the author. Together with his quest for accuracy and the ability to listen to the complaints of patients he found the underlying causes for several painful conditions of the upper extremity. It was his routine to examine not only the hand of a patient but rather to investigate the whole upper extremity and even beyond.

His tremendous experience he thus gained is laid down in this book. So he was able to explain the underlying cause of the radial and the ulnar epicondylitis as a nerve irritation of the radial and respectively the ulnar and the median nerves. Based on this he designed therapeutic measures accordingly. Of great importance is his description of the proximal radial nerve compression syndrome, where the site of compression is located at the level of the distal upper arm. Although far less common than the more distally located supinator syndrome, it may lead to frustrating results when it is missed.

The author added a major chapter to one most vexing problems of hand surgery that is the complex regional pain syndrome (CRPS), which he prefers to name after the first describer Sudeck's dystrophy. Here his routine to examine the whole upper extremity paid out when he found underlying problem being located in the area of the upper thoracic aperture. The surgical technique he described consists of decompression of the neurovascular structures in this region, combined with a decompression of the subclavian vein and an upper thoracic sympathectomy by resecting the first rib through a transaxillary approach. This procedure, which originally was designed by Ross for the treatment of resistant thoracic outlet syndrome (TOS), lead to surprisingly good results.

This present book is based upon the lifelong experience of a very busy hand surgeon. I do hope it will find the attention of the readers it deserves.

Munich, Germany   Ulrich Lanz

Preface

The monography presented here is the translation of five pain syndromes of the arm, originally published by the author in the two-volume *Hand Surgery* (ed. Towfigh et al.) of Springer Publishing Company.

The neurogenic pathogenesis of these syndromes has not been solved and proven up to now.

This concerns

- Tennis elbow (TE), with a neurogenic pathogenesis. Proof: 26 aspects, examination results, tests, and conclusions.
- Golf elbow (GE), also with a neurogenic pathogenesis. Proof: 17 aspects, examination results, tests, and conclusions.
- Proximal radial nerve compression syndrome (PRKS) in the upper arm (Wilhelm 1970). Branches of this nerve are responsible for innervation of supraepicondyle and epicondyle pain area, *namely the* collateral lateral branch of radial nerve and posterior cutaneous nerve of forearm. Whereas the posterior pain area is innervated by the anconeus muscle nerve. Proof: by aimed nerve block and surgical results.
- "So-called" coracoiditis, also with neurogenic pathogenesis. Proof: peripheral nerve-, plexus-, and stellate ganglia-blocks and surgical results of transaxillary decompression of the neurovascular bundle, including subclavian vein in TOS and SD.

A final solution of pain syndrome pathogenesis was impossible without detailed knowledge concerning the innervations of different pain areas. If these diverse surgical procedures of extensor tendon apparatus origin at the TE serve as a basis, it is shown that the positive results of these procedures depend on an automatic denervation. SD respectively CRPS I were only solved pathogenetically after the author finally discovered the "second key" in shape of a subclavian vein stenosis (1982). Pathogenesis of this dystrophy thus is based on a vascular (Wilhelm and Wilhelm 1985) and neurogenous cause (Leriche 1923).

Pathogenesis of these pain syndromes is still discussed controversially in world literature, the German titles emphasizing the surgical treatment of resistant cases were consciously changed in the sense of pathogenesis. The structure of the text, however, was not changed at all; this is also true for the order of texts, tables, and graphics.

This English monography presents the true pathogenesis of the pain syndromes mentioned to all hand-, orthopedic-, trauma-, plastic-, general- and neurosurgeons, as well as neurologists and hand-therapists of the world, together with the corresponding surgical procedures.

Furthermore this monography supports those who are interested in the two volume edition of hand surgery by Springer publishing company, but do not want, or are not able to buy it; the complete translation of which is still discussed.

Acknowledgments

At this point I want to sincerely thank my former resident Mrs. A. Christ-Günther, M.D., Ph.D., for the translation of five chapters. She undertook this project despite her family duties and her office and practice as an urologist. She always had an open ear for me.

The author also wishes to thank Dr. D. Lucas, former head of the radiological department, Klinikum Aschaffenburg, teaching hospital of Würzburg University, as well, for performing radiographic examinations and allowing their publication.

The author wishes to thank all collaborators of Springer publishing company as well who agreed with the proposal of an English translation of the pain syndromes of the arm, as already presented in 2011 in the new *Surgery of the Hand* (Towfigh et al., eds.) as a monography; main reason for this publication was the fact that all over the world the pathogenesis of these five pain syndromes is still discussed controversially, but in the meantime it has been solved and proven by the author.

- Dr. Fritz Krämer deserves a very special thank you in this context, for admitting the proposal, as well as for a long and excellent cooperation and care.
- This is also true for the editor in charge, Prof. Dr. Robert Hierner, who also admitted the proposal without any complications.
- Thanks go to Mrs. Gabriele Schroeder for informations and help
- Sincere thanks to Dr. Inga von Behrens for an excellent cooperation and eagerness to help.
- After Dr. Inga von Behrens went on vacation, her substitute Mrs. Sandra Lesny also presented with optimum cooperation and help.
- Thanks go to Mrs. Rosemarie Unger as well for her cooperation and great readiness to help.
- Thank you to Production Editors in India for preparing and correcting text, tables, and graphics, as well as bibliography.
- I am truly grateful that Prof. Ulrich Lanz wrote the *foreword* to this monography, expressing the hope, this book "will find the attention of the readers it deserves".

Summer 2014
Aschaffenburg, Germany   Albrecht Wilhelm

Contents

1   The Controversial Pain Syndrome of Tennis Elbow (TE):
Pathogenesis and Surgical Treatment of Resistant Cases   1
   1.1   Introduction   1
   1.2   Surgically Relevant Anatomy and Physiology   2
   1.3   Epidemiology   5
   1.4   Aetiology and Pathogenesis   5
   1.5   Diagnostics   16
   1.6   Classification   17
   1.7   Indications and Contraindications   17
   1.8   Therapy   18
         1.8.1   Conservative Treatment of TE   18
         1.8.2   Technique of Complete Denervation with Indirect
                  Decompression of the Deep Branch of the Radial
                  Nerve According to Wilhelm   19
         1.8.3   Postoperative Treatment   26
   1.9   Results   27
   1.10 Mistakes, Dangers and Complications   28
   References   29

2   The Controversial Pain Syndrome of GE: Pathogenesis
and Surgical Treatment of Resistant Cases   33
   2.1   Introduction   33
   2.2   Surgically Relevant Anatomy and Physiology   34
   2.3   Epidemiology   36
   2.4   Aetiology and Pathogenesis   36
   2.5   Diagnostics   44
   2.6   Classification   46
   2.7   Indications and Contraindications   46

2.8   Therapy..   46
       2.8.1   Conservative Treatment of GE   46
       2.8.2   Surgical Treatment of GE: Denervation and
               Circumcision of the Medial Epicondyle Region,
               Area According to Wilhelm   47
       2.8.3   Surgical Treatment of Resistant Cases by Denervation
               and Subcutaneous Transposition of Ulnar Nerve
               According to Wilhelm...........................   49
       2.8.4   Surgical Treatment by Additional Decompression
               of the Median Nerve at the Cubital Fossa
               According to Wilhelm...........................   51
2.9   Results...   55
2.10   Mistakes, Dangers and Complications   56
References   56

3   The Controversial Pain Syndrome of Proximal Radial
     Compression Syndrome (PRKS): Pathogenesis and Surgical
     Treatment of Resistant Cases   59
     3.1   Introduction..   59
     3.2   Surgically Relevant Anatomy and Physiology   61
     3.3   Epidemiology ,.....................................   63
     3.4   Aetiology and Pathogenesis   63
     3.5   Diagnostics   68
     3.6   Classification.......................................   69
     3.7   Therapy   71
            3.7.1   Conservative Treatment   71
            3.7.2   Surgical Treatment   71
     3.8   Results...   75
     3.9   Mistakes, Dangers and Complications   78
     References   80

4   The Controversial Pain Syndrome of the Shoulder Joint
     (So-Called Coracoiditis): Pathogenesis and Treatment
     of Resistant Cases...   83
     4.1   Introduction..   83
     4.2   Surgically Relevant Anatomy and Physiology   84
     4.3   Epidemiology   88
     4.4   Etiology and Pathogenesis   88
     4.5   Diagnostics   89
     4.6   Classification.......................................   92
     4.7   Indications and Contraindications.......................   92

4.8   Therapy..   93
       4.8.1   Technique of Partial Upper Frontal Shoulder Quadrant
               Denervation of the Shoulder Joint According
               to Wilhelm......................................   93
       4.8.2   Technique of Complete Temporary Pain Elimination
               at the Shoulder Joint According to Wilhelm..........   95
4.9   Results...   98
4.10   Mistakes, Dangers and Complications   98
References   98

5   Controversial Pain Syndrome of M. Sudeck (RSD, CRPS I):
    Pathogenesis and Surgical Treatment of Resistant Cases   101
    5.1   Introduction...   101
    5.2   Surgically Relevant Anatomy and Physiology   102
    5.3   Epidemiology   106
    5.4   Aetiology and Pathogenesis   108
    5.5   Diagnostics   111
           5.5.1   Tabular Documentation of Pathologic Findings
                   at the Upper Extremity   111
           5.5.2   Phlebography of Subclavian Vein...................   117
           5.5.3   Arteriography of Subclavian Artery   122
           5.5.4   Brachial Plexus and Intraoperative Findings   124
           5.5.5   Differential Diagnosis............................   124
    5.6   Classification..   125
    5.7   Indications and Contraindications.........................   125
    5.8   Surgical Treatment of Resistant Cases   126
           5.8.1   History...   126
           5.8.2   Informed Patient Consent   127
           5.8.3   Instruments   128
           5.8.4   Surgical Technique of Transaxillary Decompression
                   of Neurovascular Bundle and Extrapleural
                   Resection of Upper Sympathetic Trunk,
                   Respectively, Neurotomy of Communicating
                   Branches Running Towards the Lower Plexus Roots   129
    5.9   Postoperative Treatment   134
    5.10   Results...   138
    5.11   Pain Inhibitory Function of Dorsal Horn Synapsis System   143
    5.12   Mistakes, Dangers and Complications   147
    References   147

Index   151

The Controversial Pain Syndrome of Tennis Elbow (TE): Pathogenesis and Surgical Treatment of Resistant Cases

1

Contents

1.1	Introduction	1
1.2	Surgically Relevant Anatomy and Physiology	2
1.3	Epidemiology	5
1.4	Aetiology and Pathogenesis	5
1.5	Diagnostics	16
1.6	Classification	17
1.7	Indications and Contraindications	17
1.8	Therapy	18
	1.8.1 Conservative Treatment of TE	18
	1.8.2 Technique of Complete Denervation with Indirect Decompression of the Deep Branch of the Radial Nerve According to Wilhelm	19
	1.8.3 Postoperative Treatment	26
1.9	Results	27
1.10	Mistakes, Dangers and Complications	28
References		29

1.1 Introduction

The problem of tennis elbow (TE), also called epicondylitis lateralis humeri, epicondylalgia or epicondylopathy, has been known since 1834. Sir Charles Bell (ct. according to Narakas and Bonnard) described writing cramps in office employees and blamed muscle-tendon stress as the cause, due to the continuous use of a pen. Runge (1873), however, blamed a periostitis at the epicondyle extensor origins and under this aspect recommended to cut a deep scar by cauterisation. Morris (1882) detected a strain of the pronator teres muscle as cause of pain, triggered by fast and forced pronation movement of the forearm, necessary in backstroke swimming. Winckworth (1883) opposed to this opinion, remarking a strain of this muscle could hardly be responsible for all symptoms of TE.

A. Wilhelm, *Controversial Pain Syndromes of the Arm*,
DOI 10.1007/978-3-642-54513-9_1, © Springer-Verlag Berlin Heidelberg 2015

Winckworth, however, found the pain originally resulted from a pressure damage of the deep radial branch at the supinator muscle, *"where the nerve is pressed by diverse actions of the muscular fibres"*. After this first hint at a possible neurological pathogenesis of TE, this opinion was for the first time supported by Bernhart (1896), who conceived this symptom as consequence of an occupational neuralgia. Finally Major (1883) localised the origin of TE at the annular radial ligament; at the end of the nineteenth century as many as three theories of tennis elbow pathogenesis existed, namely, *the tendinogenous, neurogenous and arthrogenous theories*, a solid base for an ongoing intense discussion on aetiology and pathogenesis of this disease. Up to now, agreement was only reached concerning the primary conservative treatment of TE.

Regarding terminology, it has to be remarked that the term "epicondylitis" is misleading and incorrect, as in the area mentioned no inflammatory changes were found in case of TE (Dunkow et al. 2004; Theis et al. 2004; Faro and Wolf 2007). Also the terms epicondylalgia, epicondylopathy and supinator syndrome are not satisfactory, as diverse extents of pain in TE and the corresponding trigger points are not surveyed at all. The term tennis elbow is much better, as two essential points of this disease are characterised, namely, the aetiologically important pressure stress of the deep radial branch by acute or chronic trauma. And the second point is taking into account the fact that among diverse professions and sports, tennis players show one of the highest incidences, up to 51 % (Kipai et al. 1986, cited according to Narakas and Bonnard 1993). In only 1–3 % of the population (Goguin and Rush 2003) and among those in just about 5–10 % of patients, tennis players are found (Theis et al. 2004); still the term TE is adequate.

1.2   Surgically Relevant Anatomy and Physiology

Anatomic and clinical examinations showed the maximum pain area of TE is exclusively innervated by fibres of the radial nerve (Figs. 1.1 and 1.2).

This is also true for coincident pain areas at the back of the hand with pain radiationto the basic finger joint (*neuralgia of the posterior interosseous nerve*; Wachsmuth and Wilhelm 1967; Fig. 1.3). The coincident pain areas above the radial styloid process and in the first interosseous space, however, are innervated by branches of the superficial radial nerve. This nerve is also responsible for the dorsolateral sensibility disorder found in 19 %.

The supraepicondyle and posterior pain areas, reaching to the outer side of the elbow, are innervated by branches of the subfascial collateral lateral radial nerve branch, running behind the lateral brachial intermuscular septum and the anconeus muscle branch. The last mentioned develops from a union of the triceps muscle lateral and medial head muscular branches (Fig. 1.2), the references of which originate from the radial nerve at the upper arm, proximal to the radial nerve hiatus. The posterior antebrachii cutaneous nerve with a small branch innervates the epicondyle and the ERCB origin. Irritations of the radial nerve and its references in the region

Fig. 1.1 Typical pain area
of a severe lateral humeral
epicondylitis. Aimed
blockades can help distin-
guish individual pain areas
and their innervations. (From
Wilhelm (2000))

Puncture over the septum
intermusculare laterale for
elimination of n. cutan. antebrachii
posterior and of r. coll. ni. radialis,
with belonging pain area

Puncture for elimination
of n. radialis, with belonging
pain area

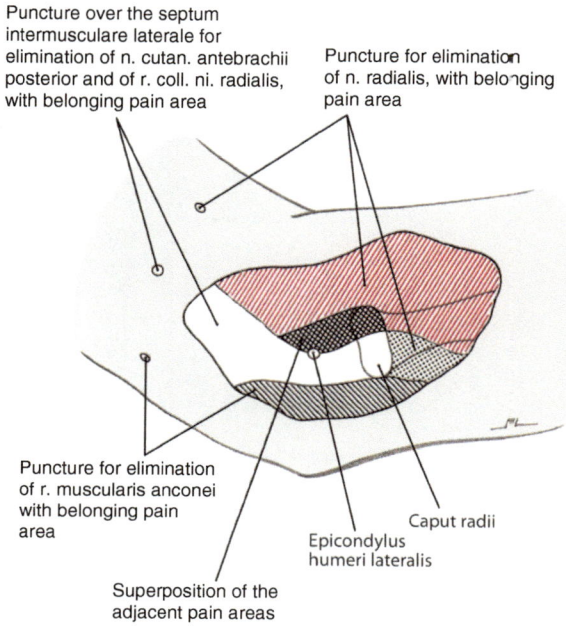

Puncture for elimination
of r. muscularis anconei
with belonging pain
area

Caput radii

Epicondylus
humeri lateralis

Superposition of the
adjacent pain areas

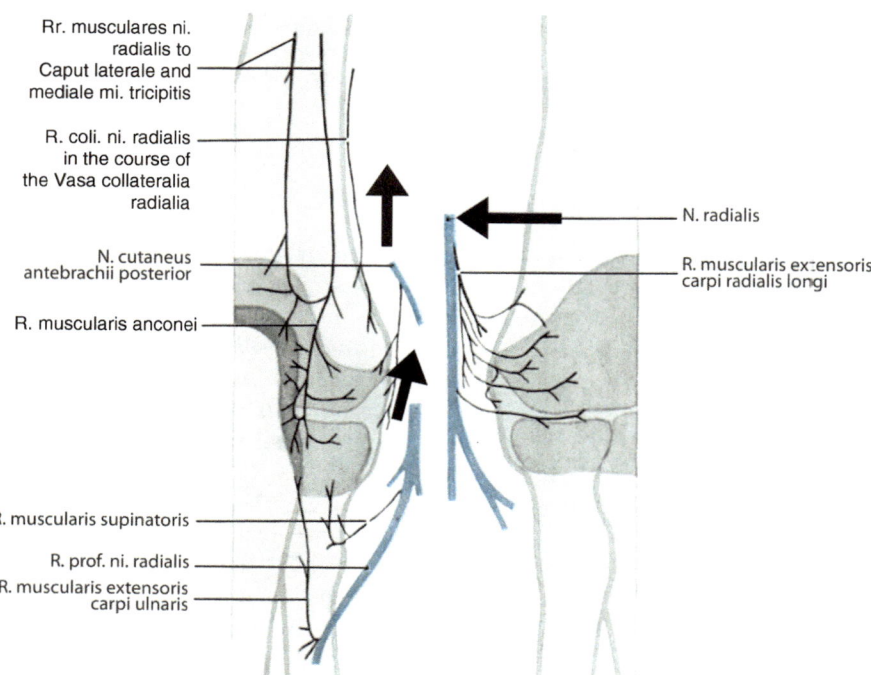

Rr. musculares ni.
radialis to
Caput laterale and
mediale mi. tricipitis

R. coli. ni. radialis
in the course of
the Vasa collateralia
radialia

N. cutaneus
antebrachii posterior

R. muscularis anconei

N. radialis

R. muscularis extensoris
carpi radialis longi

R. muscularis supinatoris

R. prof. ni. radialis
R. muscularis extensoris
carpi ulnaris

Fig. 1.2 Innervation of lateral epicondyle region from posterior (*left*) and anterior (*right*). Radial
nerve moved in lateral direction. *Black arrows*: test blockade. (According to Ishii and Nakashita
(1985)) (Taken from Wilhelm (1972))

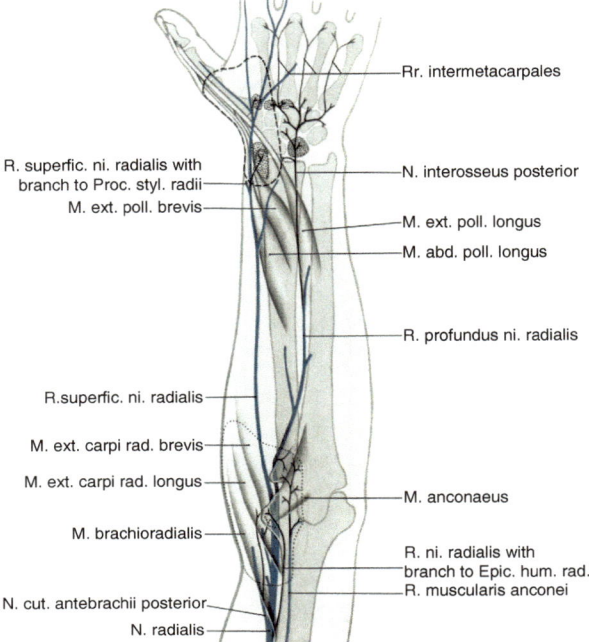

R. superfic. ni. radialis with
branch to Proc. styl. radii
M. ext. poll. brevis

R.superfic. ni. radialis

M. ext. carpi rad. brevis

M. ext. carpi rad. longus

M. brachioradialis

N. cut. antebrachii posterior

N. radialis

Rr. intermetacarpales

N. interosseus posterior

M. ext. poll. longus

M. abd. poll. longus

R. profundus ni. radialis

M. anconaeus

R. ni. radialis with
branch to Epic. hum. rad.
R. muscularis anconei

Fig. 1.3 Synopsis of irritation syndrome of radial nerve. *Punctured line*: pain area in TE. *Dotted line*: hypaesthetic zone at the superficial branch of the radial nerve. *Punctured area*: pain area in radial styloiditis. Area of intermetacarpal pain also punctured. Pain areas in neuralgia of posterior interosseous nerve above the lunate bone and base of second and third intermetacarpal bone punctured. (From Wilhelm 1972)

of the upper arm, the thoracic outlet and the intervertebral foramina C5–7 are responsible for pain manifestation in this area.

These three nerves are not involved in the original compression mechanism of the deep radial branch, but they may hint at the just mentioned areas of disturbance, possibly causing a "double nerve lesion".

• *Distally, at the extension side, an essential recurrent branch of the supinator muscle branch is found, being responsible for pain transfer in epicondyle direction. Digital pressure over the supinator gap serves as a proof.*

On the flexion side, the final muscular branch fibres of the long radial carpi extensor (ECRL) and the short radial carpi extensor (ECRB) innervate the humeroradial joint area (Fig. 1.2, right side). One of these branches (the third from above) does innervate not only the origin of ECRB tendon, where it spreads extensively, but also the epicondyle and the lateral collateral ligament. Distally a recurrent articular branch of the supinator muscle branch joins, the function of which can also be taken over by a very strong branch of the radial nerve (Fig.1.2 right side, last branch from above).

The anterior pain area extends over the epicondyle, the bulging of the radial extensors and over the course of the radial nerve, especially at the height of the humeral capitulum, the radial head and the supinator gap.

1.3   Epidemiology

The *incidence of tennis elbow* (TE) is hard to estimate, as many patients with minor complaints do not consult a physician. Generally the incidence is estimated to be 1–3 or 3–4 %, the dominant arm being affected in 90 %. The ratio male/female is 5:1. Surgical intervention due to therapy resistance is necessary in 3–8 % (Demmer and Rettig 1982). Average age of patients is between 35 and 55 years.

1.4   Aetiology and Pathogenesis

Aetiology and pathogenesis of TE are discussed controversially as of today. Since the beginning of the nineteenth century, a diversity of surgical techniques has been developed, based on different concepts of pathogenesis. The most important surgical methods are summarised in Table 1.1.

The most prominent supposition is based on functional stress together with micro-trauma and degenerative changes of tendon tissue. According to Bosworth there is an intraarticular cause of TE. Turning of the unevenly formed radial head—sometimes combined with an impingement of a synovial fold—leads to typical complaints. Recently a neurogenous genesis based on the work of Wilhelm has been discussed frequently.

The following facts and conclusions point towards a neurogenous aetiology:

1. *Anamnestic details* concerning the cause of development: sudden hyperactivity, caused by strong pronation in tennis, for example, and chronic strain of pronators and supinators as well as radial extensors, especially against resistance.
2. *Maximum extension of pain area* not only over lateral epicondyle region (Fig. 1.1).
3. *Innervation of pain area* exclusively by fibres of radial nerve (Fig. 1.2).
4. *Anatomic findings* can be proved by aimed nerve blocks, thus analysing the corresponding pain area (Fig. 1.1).
5. *A supraepicondyle and posterior pain area*, little regarded up to now, is found in 31 %, innervated by the collateral lateral branch of the radial nerve and the muscular anconeus branch, both already originating from the upper arm radial nerve (Fig 1.2).
6. The epicondyle peak and the originating tendon of ECRB are additionally innervated by fibres of the posterior antebrachii cutaneous nerve, also originating from the upper arm (Fig. 1.2). This proves that in TE also *pain radiation from farther proximal areas of radial nerve disturbance* can be expected.

Table 1.1 Surgical treatment of resistant TE – survey of literature

Author	Surgical method
Frank (1910)	Epicondylectomy
Fischer (1923)	Excision of subcutaneous tissue above epicondyle
Hohmann (1927)	Notching of ECRB tendon
Tavernier (1946)	Mononeurotomy of radial nerve lateral collateral branch
Bosworth (1955)	Partial resection of annular radial ligament
Kaplan (1959)	Partial anterior denervation
Garden (1961)	Distal lengthening of ECRB tendon
Wilhelm and Gieseler (1962)	Complete denervation
Goldie (1964)	Excision of subtendon pathologic tissue
Capener (1966)	Decompression of deep radial nerve branch
Roles and Maudsley (1972)	Decompression of radial nerve (radial tunnel)
Boyd and McLeod (1973)	Epicondylectomy and partial excision of annular radial ligament
Wilhelm (1977)	Decompression of radial nerve (upper arm)
Nirschl and Pettrone (1979)	¾ resection of ECRB tendon, release
van der Beken and Joveneau (1983)	Z-graft at ECRB and EDC
Narakas (1987)	Lengthening of ECRB and decompression of radial nerve
Wilhelm (1989)	Denervation and direct decompression of radial nerve
Wilhelm (1996, 1999, 2000)	Denervation and indirect decompression of radial nerve (method of choice since 1991)
Almquist et al. (1998)	Resection of ECRB and EDC at epicondyle–anconeus graft
Rayan et al. (2001)	V-Y graft of ECRB and EDC origins
Double nerve lesion	
Wilhelm (1996)	Transaxillar decompression of nerve-vessel bundle in TOS and Sudeck's dystrophy
Wilhelm (1977, 1996, 1999)	Decompression of radial nerve at upper arm (PRKS)

7. By *checking the trigger points of the radial nerve* at the level of the radial head in 67.8 % and above the supinator gap in 77 %, pain radiation can be triggered in the direction of the epicondyle peak and the radial nerve proximally and distally (Fig. 1.7). Analogous symptoms can be triggered by the D3 test.

8. *Coincident pain areas* of tennis elbow are found at the root of the hand, caused by neuralgia of the interosseal posterior nerve in 17.5 % (Fig. 1.3; Wachsmuth and Wilhelm 1967).

9. *Coincident sensibility disorders* are found at the superficial branch of the radial nerve in 19 %, as well as a so-called radial styloiditis in 16.7 % (Fig. 1.3).

10. *The compressive effect of the supinator arcade on the deep radial branch* can be shown by a pronation and supination test, which in 86 and 93 % absolutely tops the D3 test in 74 % (Werner 1979).

11. *Normally the supinator arcade is stretched in passive pronation*, leading to a clearly visible pressure stress of the deep radial branch (Fig. 1.4) at about 40–50 mmHg (Werner 1979). This pressure suffices to stop the intraneural venous blood flow as well as the axonal flow. Due to a coupling effect of the supinator tendon with the ECRB a tension stress of the originating tendon of this muscle, which thus shows a stretched course. *In supination, however, the*

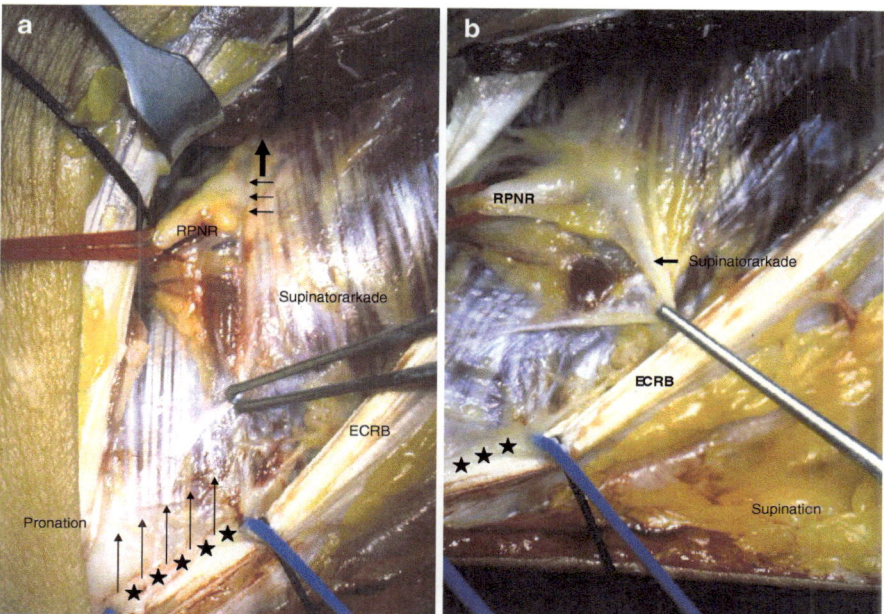

Fig. 1.4 Intraoperative presentation of supinator arcade. (**a**) In passive pronation: significant tension of the arcade and the strong superficial fascia of the supinator muscle (*thick arrow above*) with compression of the deep radial branch (RPNR) and the crossing vessels ("Henry's leash"); traction stress of ERCB tendon (*thin arrows*) by additional origin of supinator muscle from their tendon, marked by *stars* and rubber rein. (**b**) Complete relaxation of supinator muscle arcade and ERCB tendon in passive supination; no pressure stress on radial nerve

arcade and all remaining parts of the supinator muscle relax completely, as well as the ECRB tendon, then running dorsally in a more bow-shaped course (Fig. 1.4). Intraoperatively the diversity of strain stress of ERCB by the supinator arcade in pronation and supination of the forearm can be demonstrated well, slinging the additional origin of the supinator muscle proximally with a rubber rein, straining the ECRB tendon in opposite direction, where the tension stress by the rein has to remain below that of the supinator muscle (Fig. 1.4).

12. In a continuous series of 164 denervations (1980–2009) in 96.9 %, fibrous arcades of diverse strengths were found. In two cases, the arcade was situated below the deep radial branch; in three cases, it was not developed at all.

13. After direct decompression of the radial nerve (1980–1990, 87 cases), in 85 % diverse pressure damages were found. In 15 % only a disturbance of the subepineural blood flow was found (Table 1.2). But even this minor change results in an impairment of intraneural flow. Severe tension stress of the arcade can even result in major pressure damage, resulting in flattening of the nerve diameter and a bow-shaped change in the course of the nerve. Only after resection of the arcade you see the exact extent of the damage. The nervous strands stripped from the epineurium remain next to each other, but again they take a normal course (Fig. 1.5).

Table 1.2 Intraoperative findings in decompression of deep branch of radial nerve – results in group B ($N_{op}=87$)

1. *Frohse–Fränkel* arcade	
Delicate	
Structure	23 (26.4 %)
Strong	64 (73.6 %)
2. *Pressure damage of deep branch of radial nerve*	
Flattening	59 (67.8 %)
Indentation	8 (9.2 %)
Constriction ring	7 (8.0 %)
Pseudoneuroma	26 (30.0 %)
Lack of subepineural blood flow	13 (15.0 %)

14. *Two years later, these pressure damages were confirmed via electronic diagnostics; in 84%* (Kupfer et al. 1998) pathological reactions were found in EMG examinations of the forearm in neutral position as well as in passive pronation and supination (Table 1.3).

15. The immediate pain reaction in the region of origin of the common forearm extensors, triggered via D3 test, is localised in the area of the common origin of the extensor tendons by the primary description of Roles and Maudsley (1972) and is interpreted as stress of the ECRB tendon. This pain reaction can be turned off by blocking the radial nerve in the cubital fossa in 90 % (Ishii and Nakashita 1985). This surprising result negates the tendinogenous origin of this syndrome, as in this case after a blockade, still pain conduction, primarily via fibres of the posterior antebrachii cutaneous nerve would have been possible, as these innervate the lateral epicondyle and the region of origin of the ECRB tendon (Wilhelm 1999).

16. *Diverse effects of forearm positions* on the tension condition of the arcade also explain why crude strength in TE is massively reduced due to pain in pronation, at the same time being much better in supination due to a reduction of the extent of pain (Fig. 1.6). In severe pain, however, crude strength is reduced in both positions; in some cases, it cannot be measured at all. *If, preoperatively, the D3 test is negative in pronation and supination, this calls for a non-existent coupling mechanism of supinator muscle and ECRB tendon.*

17. *The compressive effect of the ligamentary arcade on the deep radial branch,* already shown in pronation, increases in this position as soon as the tendon of the ECRB is used and stressed. The cause of this phenomenon is found in an additional origin of the supinator muscle from the inner side of the tendon of origin of the ECRB (Fig. 1.7, asterisk) which has not yet been mentioned in anatomic literature. Supinator muscle and ECRB are functionally connected by the origin. Since 1991 this effect was found in 74 (91.1 %) out of 77 cases, finally explaining not only the pain reaction in D3 test but also the pathogenic significance of radial extensor overexertion, especially the ECRB. Additionally it has to be remarked that Heyse-Moore (1984) mentioned the origins of the supinator muscle and the tendon of origin of the ECRB have melted, and thus *the supinator muscle has a higher tension on the epicondyle*; this tension could

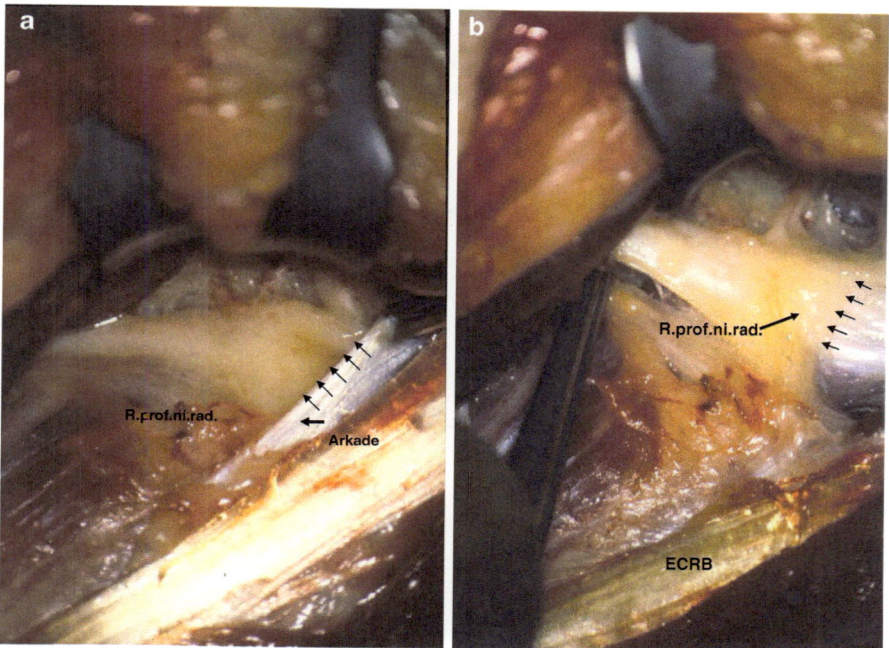

Fig. 1.5 Deep branch of radial nerve at the entrance of supinator channel (*thick arrow*). (**a**) Triple broadening of nerve diameter at the arcade under tension with thickening of epineurium (*thin arrows*). (**b**) After resection of arcade nerve fascicles lie together; the thickened epineurium has been pushed back (*thin arrows*)

Table 1.3 Development of pain level in D3 test in passive pronation and supination N; Pat. = 46 (08/04–12/07)

Pronation – EJ extended			Supination – EJ extended			Supination – EJ flexed		
n_1		%	n_2		%	N_3		%
6×	+++	13.8	20×	–	43.5	42×	–	91.3
13×	++	27.6	12×	(+)	26.0	4×	((+))	8.7
24×	+	51.7	14×	((+))	30.5			
3×	(+)	6.9						

EJ elbow joint
Pain level: extreme=+++ (VAS: 7–10); Strong=++ (VAS: 5 – 6); Intermediate=+ (VAS: 3–4); Slight=(+) (VAS: 2); Minimum=((+)) (VAS: 1); No pain=(–) (VAS: 0)

be diminished by separating the superficial head of this muscle. *Quite the contrary is the case*, however! The increased tension of the ECRB tendon, triggered as a reflex in the D3 test, leads to an increase of tension in the supinator arcade in passive pronation, due to the coupling mechanism described. Clinically this can be proven by the D3 test.

18. *D3 test is negative after denervation with indirect decompression of the radial nerve*, as in this surgical procedure a disconnection of the common origins of supinator and ECRB tendon has to be performed in order to prepare and cut the

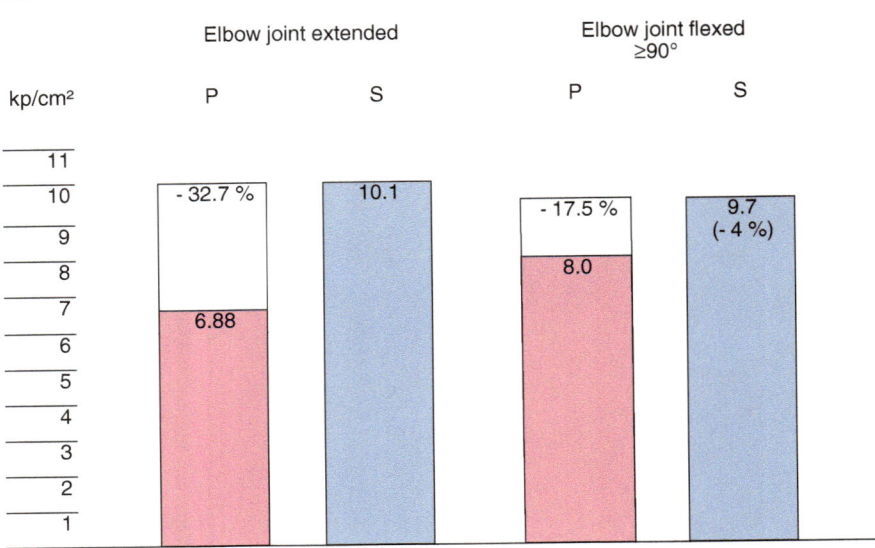

Fig. 1.6 Behaviour of crude strength in pronation (*P*) and in supination (*S*) ($N_p = 28$; 01/2007–05/2009)

anterolateral portion of origin of the supinator muscle whereby the essential pain conducting structure of the recurrent branch of the R. muscularis supinatoris is cut simultaneously (Fig. 1.7).

19. *D3 test finally turns negative in passive supination* of the forearm, in 43.5 % at simultaneous extension of the elbow joint and in 91.3 % in flexion. Minor pain remains only in 8.7 % (Table 1.3)

20. Reason being that an additional strength conduction via ECRB tendon in forearm *supination* cannot lead to results though there is a coupling mechanism, as *in this position the arcade is completely relaxed* (Fig. 1.4).

Fig. 1.7 D3-test according to Roles and Maudsley. (**a**) D3-test is performed in passive pronation of the lower arm: In D3-test there is an extensive reflectory tension of the ECRB-tendon, wherby normal tension-stress is slightly reduced by the supinator muscle. Tendon tension is so intense, however, that the coupling mechanism even results in an additional stress of the supinator-arcade, leading to an immediate pain reaction. Deep radial branch and crossing vessels are already compressed by the supinator-arcade in this position; whereas the ECRB-tendon suffers from a heightened tension-stress by the coupling mechanism, described. (**b**) D3-test in pronation: In this case we can find a typical radiation of pain to the lateral epicondyle and in proximal and distal direction of the radial nerve, *s. arrow*; supinator cleft: *s. ring with asterisk*. (**c**) Position in passive supination: Due to the slackening of the supinator muscle and its arcarde the effect of the above mentioned coupling mechanism does not work in supination. (**d**) D3-test in passive supination: In this position supinator muscle and its arcade are completely relaxed, whereby the pain is reduced clearly

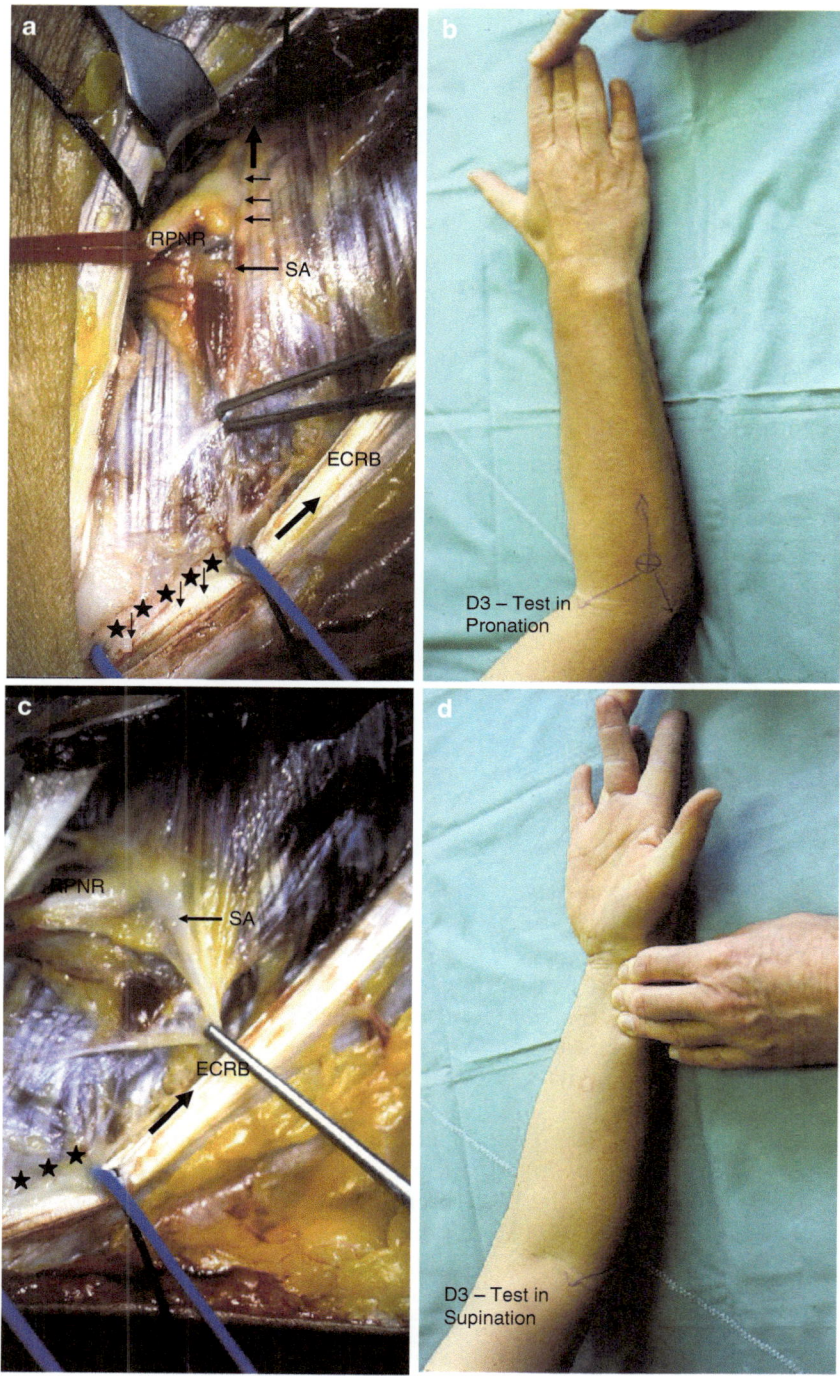

Table 1.4 Tennis elbow in proximal compression of radial nerve (PRKS) results after decompression (1969–1988: $N_p = 13 - N_{op} = 13$)

Preoperative findings	n	Postoperative results	
		Excellent	No change
Pain regions			
Epicondyle region	13	9	2 (+2)
Neuralgia of posterior interosseous nerve	5	3	1 (+1)
Radial styloiditis	4	3	0 (+1)
Sensibility disorders (superficial branch of radial nerve)	19	16	2 (+1)

Results in brackets based on an independent "radial tunnel syndrome" by Roles and Maudsley

Table 1.5 *Tennis elbow in T. O. S. (1982–1987: $N_p = 92$ – follow-ups: $N_{op} = 100$)*

Preoperative findings	n	Postoperative results			
		Excellent	Good	Fair	No change
Tennis elbow	86	48	17	7	14
Radial tunnel, proximal section	8	4	–	2	2
Radial tunnel, medial section	34	14	4	8	8
Radial tunnel, distal section	29	21	1	3	4
Neuralgia of posterior interosseous nerve	22	18	–	1	3
Radial styloiditis	18	11	1	3	3
Sensibility disorders (superficial branch of the radial nerve)	9	4	–	5	–
Total	206 (100 %)	120 (58.3 %)	23 (11.2 %)	29 (14.0 %)	34 (16.5 %)

21. TE has a special meaning in a so-called double nerve lesion. Thus in PRKS according to Wilhelm (1999), surgical decompression of the radial nerve at the upper arm showed excellent and good results in 9 (69 %) out of 13 cases (Table 1.4). Also surgical treatment of an overlying TOS as well as Sudeck's dystrophy in 65 (76 %) out of 86 cases (Table 1.5) and in 7 (70 %) out of 10 cases showed significant improvement of classical TE symptoms (Table 5.3; Wilhelm 1996). The intervertebral foramina C5–C7 can also cause a double nerve lesion.

22. *The excellent and good results of this surgical procedure of choice in approximately 93% support the neurogenous pathogenesis of TE* (Wilhelm 1999, 2000; Tables 1.6, 1.7, and 1.8). This rating also took into account the results of a postoperative check of chair, D3 and PS test, as well as crude strength, also in comparison of both sides (Tables 1.9 and 1.10). These results were already confirmed in an early compilation of statistics. Excellent and good results in 90–92 % were found in 356 (50 %) out of 711 surgical procedures. In 355 (50 %) surgical procedures results ranged 80–88 % (Wilhelm 1999).

23. *These results* were accomplished without incision, excision, resection or Z and V-Y plastic of the extensor tendons; they *were reached solely by combination*

Table 1.6 Modified evaluation system according to Roles and Maudsley

1 (excellent)	No pain, free motion, full activity range and reconstitution of crude strength
2 (good)	Rare complaints, free motion, full activity range and reconstitution of crude strength
3 (fair)	Pain after longer exertion; mild pressure pain at radial nerve and/or its deep branch, distant pain; subjectively definitely improved since surgery, reduction of crude strength
4 (poor)	No improvement

Table 1.7 Techniques of denervation (groups A, B and C_{I+II}) – follow-up

	A. Denervation (1970–1990)	B. Denervation and direct decompression of the deep branch of radial nerve (1980–1990)	C. Denervation and indirect decompression of the deep branch of radial nerve	
			C_I (1991–1994)	C_{II} (1996–2009)
Patients	39	81	46	31
Followed up	36 (92.3 %)	69 (85.2 %)	42 (91.3 %)	28 (90.3 %)
Operations	39	87	46	31
Followed up	36 (92.3%)	75 (86.2 %)	42 (91.3 %)	28 (90.3 %)

of denervation with indirect decompression of the deep radial branch after primary dissolution of the coupling mechanism of supinator muscle and ECRB. The incision of the supinator muscle anterior and lateral portions of origin at the level of the distal radial head rim, necessary for denervation of the recurrent supinator branch, also leads to an indirect decompression of the deep radial branch and results in much better postoperative results. Consequently the former technique of denervation with direct decompression of the nerve was left (Table 1.8, group B and C1/2).

24. As a consequence TE pathogenetically only is the result of radial nerve pressure damage, its originating fibres and branches, whereby nerve irritations triggering pain can be found at one or more localisations. The supinator gap syndrome (TE) is second to the carpal tunnel syndrome in nerve compression syndromes of the upper extremity.

25. To sum up, it can be said, the tendinogenous pathogenesis of TE as still discussed today is not as important as formerly thought. Under this aspect, the causal degenerative development at the extensors should only be discussed as a coincidence, even more as the TE frequency peak is about 10 years prior to degeneration of tendons (Goldie 1964).

26. If diverse surgical sections in procedures at the extensor tendon apparatus are based on the innervation of the entire pain area in TE, it is found that the success of these procedures, whatever you do, is based on a partial to complete denervation and in most excellent cases in an unconscious relaxation of the supinator arcade.

The following examples are judged epicritically: The good results of the Hohmann technique can only be achieved by deep incision of the ECRB tendon, the stumps "afterwards gape by 1 cm" (Hohmann 1949). Visualising the flow of procedures in this method topographically anatomically, it is shown that in preparation of

Table 1.8 Postoperative results – evaluation

Group	A (1970–1990)		B (1980–1990)		C$_I$ (1991–1994)		C$_{II}$ (1996–2009)	
Excellent	29 (80.5 %)	(91.6 %)	36 (48.0 %)	(65.3 %)	33 (78.6 %)	(90.5 %)	21 (75.0 %)	(92.9 %)
Good	4 (11.1 %)		13 (17.3 %)		5 (11.9 %)		5 (17.9 %)	
Fair	2 (5.6 %)		16 (21.3 %)		3 (7.1 %)		2 (7.1 %)	
Poor	1 (2.8 %)		10 (13.4 %)		1 (2.4 %)		0 (0.0 %)	
Follow-up (years)	9.7		3.6		7.3		3.5	
Disablement (weeks)	2.7		11.7		5.7		5.9	

After modified system according to Roles and Maudsley (1972)

Table 1.9   Denervation results including function tests – patient population: 1991–1994

Sex: 19 M: 23 F
Age: 43.92 (22.58–62.14) years
Localisation: dominant side (32×) subordinate side (10×)

Evaluation	n (42/46)	Chair test	D3 test	PS test
1 = Excellent	32 (76.2 %)	32 × o. B.	32 × o. B.	32 × o. B.
2 = Good	7 (16.6 %)	5 × o. B.	5 × o. B.	5 × o. B.
		2 × ((+))	2 × ((+))	2 × ((+))
3 = Fair	2 (4.8 %)	1 × o. B.	1 × (+)	1 × o. B.
		1 × (+)	1 × ((+))	1 × ((+))
4 = Poor	1 (2.4 %)	1 × +	1 × +	1 × +

Follow-up: 7.3 (5.25–9.0) years/disablement 5.7 (1.0–9.6) weeks
Pain degree: no pain = o. B., minimal = ((+)) (VAS: 1); slight = (+) (VAS: 2); medium = + (VAS: 3 – 4)

Table 1.10   Postoperative evaluation of crude strength in groups with excellent and good results ($n = 25$ and 9) – patient population 1970–1990

Sex M/F	n (25/39)	Operations dominant side $P = kp/cm^2$ $S =$ side difference (%)	n (9/39)	Operations subordinate side $P = kp/cm^2$ $S =$ side difference (%)
M	13	$P = 0.90$ (0.76 bis 1.23) $S = 5.95$ (−4.7 bis 20.0)	4	$P = 0.78$ (0.56 bis 1.18) $S = 3.60$ (−3.4 bis 8.9)
F	12	$P = 0.72$ (0.52 bis 0.94) $S = 15.95$ (−3.7 bis 28.5)	5	$P = 0.65$ (0.56 bis 0.90) $S = 4.8$ (−6.7 bis 11.4)

Remark: due to time and financial reasons 5 (12.4 %) out of 39 patients were only checked by telephone call

the epicondyle and the extensor tendon plate unconsciously, a cut of the most important final cutaneous antebrachii posterior nerve branch fibres is performed; final fibres of muscular branches of ECRL can also be incised. The essential part is an unconscious additional incision of the supinator origin, *whereby the recurrent nerve branch of the supinator muscle is cut simultaneously*; *only then the stumps of the ECRB tendon can gape.*

Similar thoughts apply to the surgical techniques of Bosworth (1955), Goldie (1964), Boyd and McLeod (1973), Nirschl and Pettrone (1979), van der Beken and Joveneau (1983) and Rayan et al. (2001).

The procedure according to Almquist et al. (1998) *is the only one, the results of which are based on a nearly complete unconscious denervation.* Only the collateral lateral branch of the radial nerve, running behind the lateral intermuscular septum of the arm and only innervating the supraepicondyle pain area is not cut. By resection of the common origins of the extensor tendons down to the articular capsule and the lateral ligament also, the essential pain conducting nerve, being the recurrent fibre of the supinator muscle branch, is cut and the supinator arcade is relaxed, that is, the deep branch of the radial nerve is decompressed. The elimination of the proximally spreading muscular anconeus branch final fibres was accomplished unconsciously by covering the defect of the extensor tendon with transfer of the anconeus muscle. This nerve, by the way, is neither mentioned in the text nor depicted. Relating to the innervation of this muscle, there are only hints at a nerve-vessel strand distally entering the muscle. Good results in 62–87 % are based on the extent of resection and on the combination with an anconeus plastic.

- *Solving the pathogenesis of TE lead to the acknowledgement of occupational cooperatives concerning financial demands regarding an occupational sickness in professions focusing on an overexertion of pronation and supination movements against resistance.*

1.5   Diagnostics

Symptoms of TE arise from a sudden event or from chronic overexertion of pronators and supinators as well as radial extensors, also in combination with flexion and extension in the elbow joint. This is especially true in extensive development of force and resistance, for example, in construction, metal and wood workers.

This symptom can also develop in jobs demanding extremely quick finger movements, such as musicians and secretaries. In this context one has to inquire about shoulder, arm and hand pain as well as the sitting position at work. Knowledge of toxic influences, of metabolic and inflammatory diseases as well as of focal toxic lesions, especially focused on teeth, tonsils and paranasal sinus, as well as abdominal organs, is essential, in order to prevent the danger of an irritating increase in nervous structures, an increase in scarring and a focal arthritis by a pretreatment.

After surgery of a *chronic tonsillitis*, it is frequently seen that TE symptoms subside after a few days. Further pathogenic connections of this *phenomenon* cannot be explained yet.

In judging TE an overlying irritation of the radial nerve and its relations at the upper arm (PRKS), the thoracic outlet and the intervertebral foramina (C5–C7) should not be overlooked. Findings of this examination have to be documented as well. This also applies to coincident pain areas of the hand, caused by a neuralgia of the posterior interosseous nerve, for sensibility disturbances in the area of the posterior cutaneous antebrachii nerve and the superficial branch of the radial nerve with corresponding radial styloiditis.

Next, palpation determines the entire pain area of TE, *focusing not only on the epicondyle* but also on the area of the radial extensors and the course of the radial nerve in the elbow and the supinator channel, further on the supraepicondyle pain area, innervated by the collateral lateral branch of the radial nerve and the posterior antebrachii cutaneous nerve, reaching as far as up to the outer side of the olecranon (posterior pain area). The muscular branch of the anconeus innervates this area (Fig. 1.2).

Palpation of the brachial plexus follows, as well as palpation of pain localisations at the shoulder joint and diverse sections of the radial channel, checking sensibility disorders of the lateral cutaneous brachii nerve, the posterior cutaneous antebrachii nerve and the superficial branch of the radial nerve. *A neuralgia of the posterior interosseous nerve* (Wachsmuth and Wilhelm 1967) *is checked by the hand joint flexion test* leading to an increase of traction of the interosseous nerve, answered by a corresponding triggering of pain. The test can also be positive in irritation distal to the supinator gap or further proximally. *Palpation of the supinator gap* is essential for diagnosis, as it triggers pain radiation at the radial nerve proximally and distally, but especially in the direction of the epicondyle, patients report and demonstrate them frequently (Fig. 1.7). Especially this finding is a further proof of TE's neurogenous pathogenesis.

Results of crude strength and D3 test should be checked not only in passive pronation (Fig. 1.7) *but also in passive supination* (Fig. 1.7) in extended and flexed elbow joint (>90°). The strength and pain values of this exam should be rated in points according to VAS and should also be documented in tables (Fig. 1.6, Table 1.3).

The pronation and supination test against resistance according to Werner (1979) is important as its results top the D3 test, and it also demonstrates the compressive effect of the supinator arcade on the deep radial branch.

In *differential diagnosis* arthrogenous diseases and results of accidents have to be ruled out. Basic diagnostics of an elbow-joint x-ray in two levels suffices. Should this not be sufficient, an arthroscopy has to be performed. Suspicion of a rupture at the extensor tendon origin needs ultrasound examination. In unclear findings NMR is necessary, as well as in suspicion of bursitis and development of a deeper tumour, especially in painful AV fistula, osteofibroma and glomus tumour. Radiologic and neurologic exams have to analyse radicular disturbances. In differential diagnosis you also find TOS and an early stage of Sudeck's dystrophy which can only be diagnosed or ruled out in systematically examining the entire upper extremity and in documenting pathologic findings (Fig. 5.7).

For forensic reasons a neurologic exam is also necessary to further support the diagnosis. *An examination according to* Kupfer et al. (1998) *is necessary*, as earlier examinations in central position of the forearm showed corresponding pathologic findings in only 5–10 %, which from today's point of view added to the insecurity of TE pathogenesis.

1.6 Classification

Due to therapeutic reasons, TE should be classified into an acute form, resistant to conservative therapy, and a chronic recurrent form.

1.7 Indications and Contraindications

All over the world there is an agreement upon primarily treating acute TE conservatively. It has to be taken into account that symptoms, even in severe disease, can vanish completely within 6 months by convalescent treatment and ban of the triggering factor (occupational pause, no tennis, etc.), as well as by application of simple pain killers.

In therapy-resistant cases despite additional treatment, *indication for denervation with indirect decompression of the deep radial branch* is given; this is also true in chronic recurrent disease. If there is no posterior pain area, an additional cutting of the anconeus muscular branch final fibres by temporary loosening of the distal triceps fibres and the origin of the anconeus muscle is not necessary, as long as the patient does not belong to certain occupational groups, for instance, carrying heavy loads in flexed elbow joint position or working heavily with extreme strain of pronator and supinator muscles against resistance, even using the triceps muscles. These conditions lead to pain radiation into the posterior pain area by irritation of the radial nerve at the upper arm via the nerve branch of the anconeus muscle.

Focus should be on secretaries and musicians using fingers quickly mainly in pronation of the forearm, as in strings with the bow arm and in piano players even on both sides. Sometimes complete denervation is necessary in these and similar cases of a posterior pain area are found.

Contraindications are given if there is suspicion of a focal toxic process which first has to be analysed and treated, further on in overlying disturbances such as neurologically verified PRKS, TOS or Sudeck's dystrophy. If there is suspicion of a foramen stenosis, a neurological exam is essential as radicular disturbances have to be ruled out. The indication for TE surgery in this case should also be discussed with the neurologist.

In a clear PRKS with hypaesthesia at the inferior lateral brachial cutaneous nerve and the posterior antebrachial cutaneous nerve, surgery of TE should not be the first step of treatment, as after decompression of the radial nerve at the upper arm in 9 (81.8 %) out of 11 cases symptoms of TE are not found any more (Table 1.4). Also in TOS TE should not primarily be treated surgically, but one should wait for the success of conservative or surgical treatment of this syndrome. After this procedure vanishing of TE symptoms can be expected in about 75.6 % (Table 1.5). TE in Sudeck's dystrophy must not primarily be operated due to danger of deterioration of dystrophic conditions with increase of VAS values. In this case improvement after successful conservative and surgical treatment is 80 % (Table 5.3).

1.8   Therapy

1.8.1   Conservative Treatment of TE

An immediate elimination or change of anamnestically possible causes stands at the start of *conservative treatment* in any case, as this disease is based on neurologic causes as an occupational neuralgia (Winckworth 1883, Bernhart 1896). These causes can be found in occupational as well as in recreational activities, as playing tennis, for example.

Basic treatment in acute and very painful start of symptoms are non-exertion with avoidance of pronation and an analgetic and anti-inflammatory therapy is most important. In these cases, injection of a long-lasting anaesthetic about two fingerbreadths below the radial head has been successful. Thereby the essential recurrent supinator branch is eliminated. Blockade of the deep radial branch is accomplished by diffusion. *A combination with a corticosteroid is not recommended* any more, due to well-known side effects up to humeroradial capsule defects.

- *The only specific conservative treatment of TE is the immobilisation of the arm in supination of the forearm by a well-padded detachable plastic cast for the upper arm.*

Only in this position a complete relaxation of the supinator muscle including its arcade can be reached, resulting in a complete pressure relief of the deep radial branch with consecutive normalisation of blood flow and intraneural flow. Shoulder and finger joints can be moved immediately as in supination the mentioned coupling effect cannot develop at all. Valium and elevated positioning of the arm in abduction without inner rotation are recommended. Time of immobilisation depends on local findings and strength of pain. In swelling of soft tissue, the dressing has to be checked first and possibly has to be reapplied more loosely. Discontinuation of immobilisation during daytime should be accompanied by a physiotherapist.

Immobilisation of the arm in supination can also be attempted in chronic recurring tennis elbow, also in order to convince the patient of the success of treatment and to render the agreement in a denervation with indirect decompression of the deep radial branch easier.

In a survey it was shown that in treatment phase level 1 "monotherapy…only shows evidence of a clinically relevant effect up to the sixth week after start of treatment" (Theis et al. 2004). After this, only a placebo effect is found. This especially concerns the use of NSA, infiltration anaesthetics and local corticosteroid injections combined with local anaesthetics and also physical and physiotherapy as well as the so-called epicondyle braces and wrist splints to relax the radial extensors. Also there were no advantages by treatment via ultrasound and electric stimulation (Rineer and Rush 2009).

There are diverse opinions concerning *extracorporeal lithotriptors* (ESWT). Rompe et al. (1996) report an improvement of pain and function after 1 year in 48 % compared to 30 % in the control group. After checking nine series of trials with over 1,000 patients, Buchbinder et al. (2005) concluded that ESWT had no special effect.

1.8.2 Technique of Complete Denervation with Indirect Decompression of the Deep Branch of the Radial Nerve According to Wilhelm

1.8.2.1 Informed Patient Consent
- Explanation of surgical principle and possible combined procedures, like arthrotomies and/or revisions of nerve in relapse surgery:
- Duration of surgery approximately 45–60 min, up to 1 h longer in relapse surgery
- Success rate over 90 %
- Common postoperative complications as infection, bleeding, swelling of soft tissue, etc.

- Remaining complaints, especially in independently remaining areas of disturbance at the upper arm, shoulder, neck and upper spine area
- Possibility of a transient nerve damage in revision procedures
- Ugly scar
- Limitation of elbow motion (rare)
- Sudeck's dystrophy; not found in own patient population
    - *Usually 1–3 % of surgically treated TE need a complete decompression of the deep radial branch in a second session; thus it is advisable to inform the patient at the end of the conversation.*
- For optimum approach between ECRB and EDC according to Guild and Stookey (1919; cit. according to Henry 1973), only a lengthening of the prior incision is necessary (Figs. 1.8 and 1.9). In these cases as well, a preoperative neurological exam should be performed.

1.8.2.2 Instruments
- Instruments for hand surgery
- Fine electric knife
- Magnifying glasses in revision of radial nerve

1.8.2.3 Anaesthesia and Positioning
- Intubation
- Upper or lower plexus anaesthesia and intravenous, regional anaesthesia
- Position on the back
- Bandaging of the upper arm towards the trunk and application of a controlled upper arm deprivation of blood supply, cuff 200–300 mmHg
- Positioning of slightly flexed elbow joint on a cloth padding

1.8.2.4 Skin Incision
After preparing the area of surgery, the supraepicondyle crista, the epicondyle peak and the radial head are determined and marked for orientation in the skin incision. Preparation of the lateral epicondyle region by a posterior bow-shaped circumcision

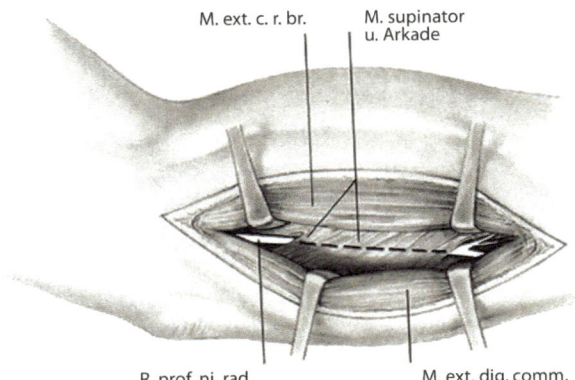

Fig. 1.8 Preparation of radial nerve deep branch in the supinator-channel according to Guild and Stookey. (From Wilhelm (1986), with kind permission of Thieme)

M. ext. c. r. br.   M. supinator u. Arkade

R. prof. ni. rad.   M. ext. dig. comm.

Fig. 1.9 Status post complete decompression of deep radial branch. The lateroposterior half of the superficial head (below) is resected. There are altogether four compressive areas with interruption of the subepineural course of the vessel, marked by *arrows*. The most severe pressure damage in this case happened at the exit of the supinator channel (right side, below); here the epineurium has been pushed back (cf. Fig. 1.5)

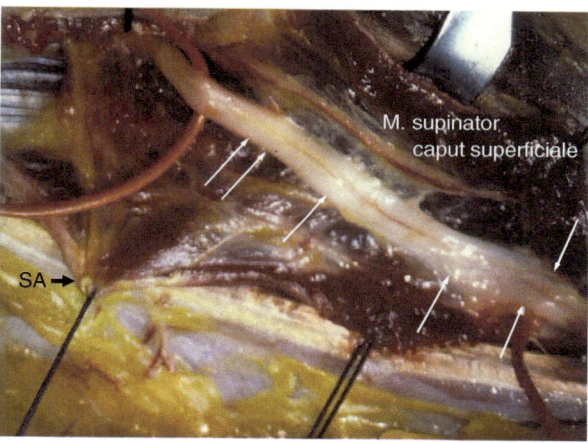

of the epicondyle (Fig. 1.10). The incision starts 4–5 cm above the epicondyle, directly behind the palpable epicondyle crista, ending 2–3 cm distal to the radial head. Lengthening of the approach (hatched line) is only indicated in relapse procedures in order to prepare the radial nerve and its branches. In preparation of the subcutaneous tissue, branches of the posterior antebrachii cutaneous nerve have to be spared, as one of them might also run behind the crista as an exception. *Anterior cuts should not be performed* in order to keep branches of this nerve out of danger.

Presentation of the lateral collateral nerve-vessel strand at the upper arm.

The proximal epifascial preparation of soft tissue is performed up to above the ECRL origin and distally 2–3 cm below the radial head.

By loosening the anterior soft tissue coat, delicate nerve endings of the posterior antebrachii cutaneous nerve are already cut blindly.

The longitudinal incision of the fascia is performed directly above the supraepicondyle crista up to the epicondyle peak presenting the lateral collateral nerve-vessel bundle running directly behind the lateral intermuscular septum. These structures are incised electrically at the proximal angle of the wound (left arrow) onto the rim in transverse direction, cutting supraepicondyle pain up to the cranial base of the epicondyle (Fig. 1.11).

Anterior pain area: Loosening ECRL and separating the portions of origin of both radial extensors.

After angle-shaped lengthening of the fascial incision between the well recognisable radial extensors follows, the loosening and isolation of the ECRL with an electric knife, cutting around the anterior circumference of the epicondyle, diligently dissecting the anterior humerolateral joint capsule first up to the height of the radial head. The anterior intra- and extramuscular end fibres of the radial nerve running to the epicondyle and innervating a part of the tendon of origin of the ECRB (Fig. 1.12) are cut. In order to be sure, the periosteum at the joint capsule is incised with an electric knife. Then the anterior and lateral portion of origin of the supinator muscle is shown in pronation of the forearm. Here both radial extensors need to be

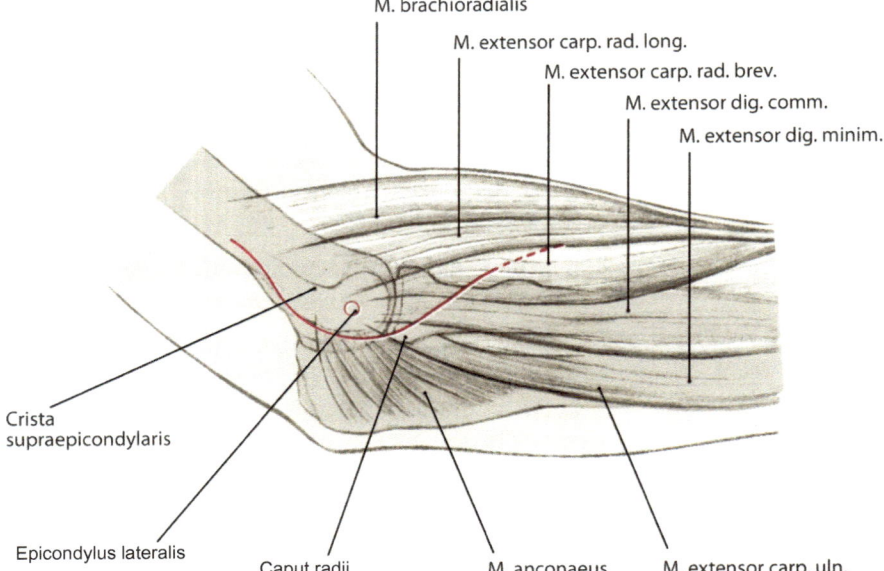

M. brachioradialis

M. extensor carp. rad. long.

M. extensor carp. rad. brev.

M. extensor dig. comm.

M. extensor dig. minim.

Crista
supraepicondylaris

Epicondylus lateralis

Caput radii

M. anconaeus

M. extensor carp. uln.

Fig. 1.10 Posterior incision around the lateral humeral epicondyle; lengthening of incision in revision procedure hatched in *red*. (From Wilhelm (2000), with kind permission of Urban and Vogel)

separated 2–3 cm further distally in order to check the radial head and neck exactly. After prior incision of the superficial fascia, the division of the muscle fibres is accomplished bluntly by using a curved clamp; in the depth you reach a strong common radial extensor plate of origin, being resected at the rim after longitudinal incision proximally, in order to prevent extreme scarring.

Dissection has to be performed in pronation of the forearm in order to definitely prevent lesion of the deep radial branch.

In this position the nerve runs 4–6 cm distal to the humeroradial joint (Figs. 1.12 and 1.13).

Cutting off the recurrent supinator muscle branch and dissolving the coupling mechanism (Fig. 1.14): The essential part of denervation starts with an isolated presentation of the anterior and lateral supinator muscle portion of origin. Here the prior hardly recognised additional origin of the supinator muscle is loosened from the inner side of the ECRB tendon (Fig. 1.4, marked by asterisk and a blue rubber band). Afterwards this portion of origin is distally either leashed (Fig. 1.4) or positioned above a curved clamp and then cut (Fig. 1.15), also at the same time dissolving the coupling mechanism mentioned. Only then the supinator muscle anterior and lateral portions of origin can be presented clearly (Figs. 1.16 and 1.17) and can be incised above the distal rim of the radial head (Figs. 1.18 and 1.19) in order to cut off the pain leading recurrent fibres of the supinator muscle branch. A gap of 6–8 mm remains in the anterior wound area of the superficial supinator head, completely

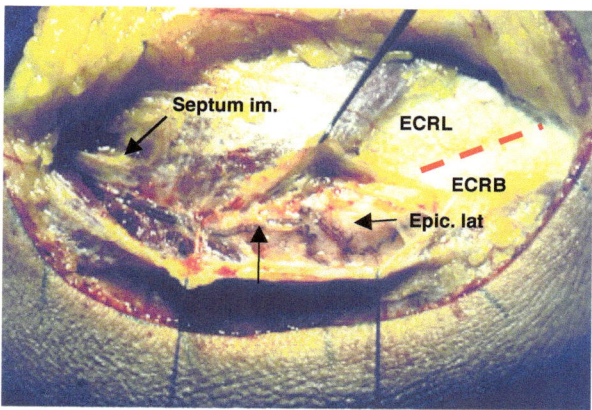

Fig. 1.11 Status post epifascial loosening of anterior soft tissue coat. The posterior antebrachii cutaneous nerve is not seen in the subcutaneous fatty tissue. Status post incision of superficial fascia directly below the lateral intermuscular septum. The lateral collateral nerve-vessel bundle is isolated then. The course of thin final fibres of the collateral nerve branch can only be seen indirectly by the covering fatty structures (*small arrow*). The transverse incision of the nerve-vessel bundle happens behind the septum at the *arrow* (left above) up to the supraepicondyle crista. Then septum and ECRL are loosened directly at the humerus up to the epicondyle peak. Lengthening of fascia incision to separate both radial extensors is hatched in *red*

sufficient to relax this part of the muscle and its arcade and at the same time entirely relaxing the deep radial branch.

Posterior pain area: *Cutting off the final fibres of the muscular branch of the anconeus.*

Next the nerve supply of the posterior pain area (Fig. 1.2) via delicate fibres of the muscular anconeus branch is cut. First the superficial fascia between ulnar carpi extensor muscle and anconeus muscle has to be lengthened from the epicondyle peak in distal direction. Then the distal fibres of the triceps are cut from the distal humerus by electric knife, whereas the anconeus muscle is cut at its origin and flapped back diligently saving the posterior articular capsule (Fig. 1.12).

Drainage, wound closure, dressing and immobilisation (Fig. 1.20).

After opening the partial deprivation of blood supply, diligent control of haemorrhage and application of a Redon drainage into the frontal wound area, first the anconeus muscle is reinserted with absorbable suture (figure of eight suture). Afterwards reinsertion of the remaining muscles is performed by a continuous suture of the opposite fascial rims, also with absorbable suture 4/0, *with exception of the supinator muscle*. After closing the wound, the compressive dressing is applied, reaching from the middle of the hand to the upper arm; the immobilisation of the elbow joint is accomplished in slight flexion (0-30-0), middle position of the forearm and slight extension of the wrist (0-20-0) by a dorsal upper arm plastic cast.

Fig. 1.12 Status post loosening the ECRL up to the frontal articular capsule and separating both radial extensors. Status post cutting the collateral nerve-vessel bundle marked by *arrow*. In the posterior area status post loosening distal triceps fibres and anconeus muscle. (From Wilhelm (2000), with kind permission of Urban and Vogel)

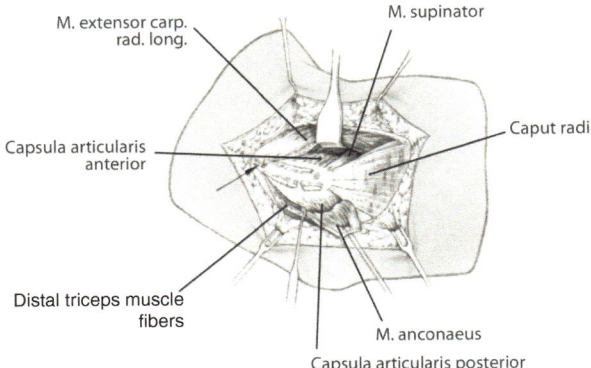

M. extensor carp. rad. long.

M. supinator

Caput radii

Capsula articularis anterior

Distal triceps muscle fibers

M. anconaeus

Capsula articularis posterior

Fig. 1.13 Status post separation of both radial extensors with preparation of the arcade, the deep branch of radial nerve and the crossing bundle of vessels, which must not be resected in order to protect the nerve gliding bed

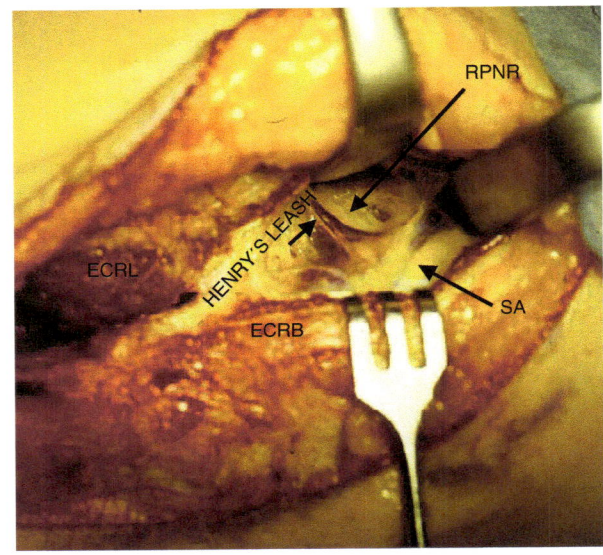

RPNR

ECRL

HENRY'S LEASH

ECRB

SA

Fig. 1.14 Additional origin of supinator muscle from ECRB marked by line punctured in *red*. Later incision of supinator muscle above the distal rim of the radial head, accentuated by *red curved line*. (From Wilhelm (2000), with kind permission of Urban and Vogel)

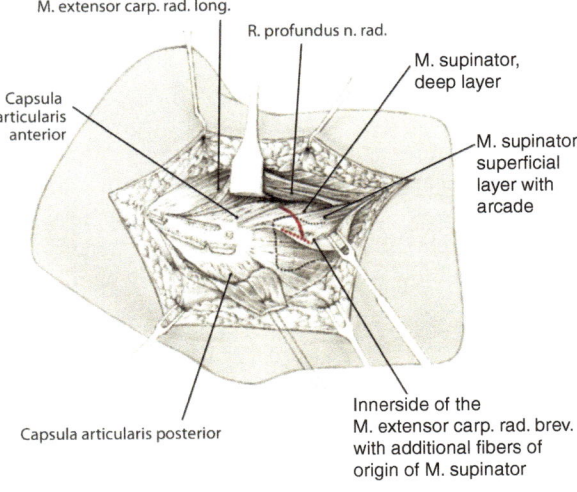

M. extensor carp. rad. long.

R. profundus n. rad.

M. supinator, deep layer

Capsula articularis anterior

M. supinator, superficial layer with arcade

Capsula articularis posterior

Innerside of the M. extensor carp. rad. brev. with additional fibers of origin of M. supinator

Fig. 1.15 Moving below additional supinator origin from the inner side of the ECRB, incision line marked by *asterisks*. *RPNR* radius profundus ni. radialis

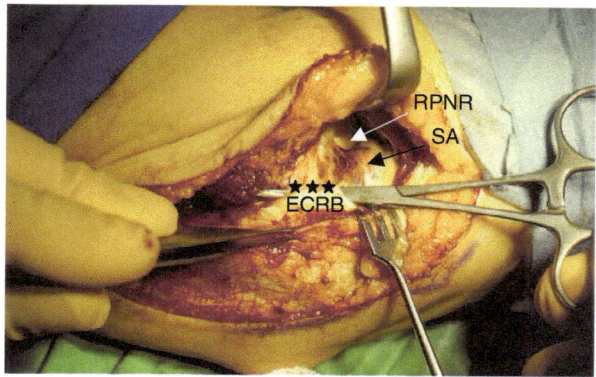

Fig. 1.16 Status post discontinuation of coupling between supinator muscle and ECRB. Incision height of anterolateral portion of origin of supinator muscle marked by *red line*. As all surgical steps in this area have to be performed in pronation the arcade is stretched, compressing nerves, four *short arrows*, *long arrow* tension of the arcade by pronation. For didactic reasons crossing vessels (Fig. 1.13) were omitted. (From Wilhelm (2000), with kind permission of Urban and Vogel)

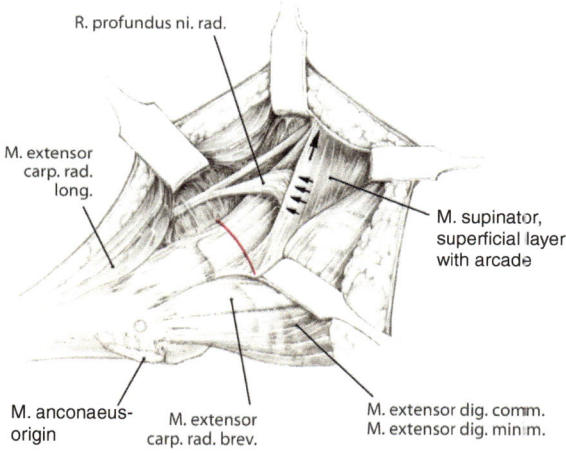

Fig. 1.17 Status post discontinuation of coupling, base gripped by forceps, *SA* supinator arcade, *black arrow*

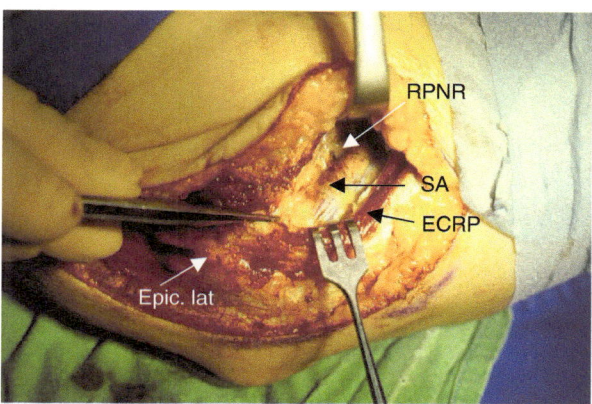

Fig. 1.18 Status post discontinuation of coupling and incision of supinator muscle anterolateral portion of origin (*red band*). Arcade is relaxed and deep radial branch is not compressed any more. (From Wilhelm (2000), with kind permission of Urban and Vogel)

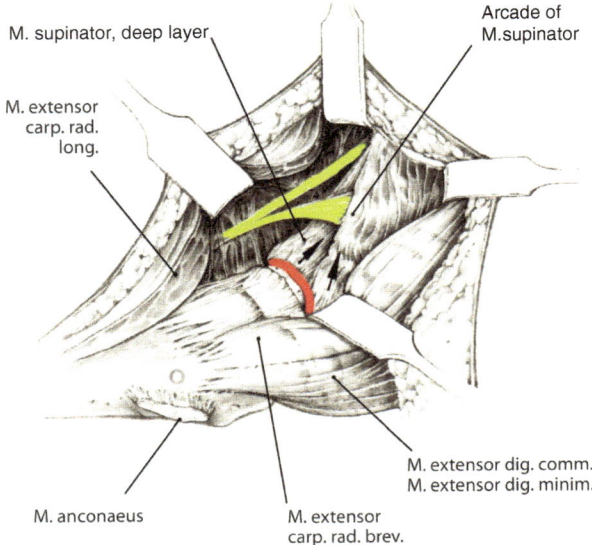

M. supinator, deep layer

Arcade of M.supinator

M. extensor carp. rad. long.

M. anconaeus

M. extensor carp. rad. brev.

M. extensor dig. comm.
M. extensor dig. minim.

Fig. 1.19 Status post cutting supinator muscle anterolateral portion of origin (*double headed arrow*). Distinct diastasis of muscle stumps and relaxation of arcade, *RPNR* radius ptofundus ni. radialis

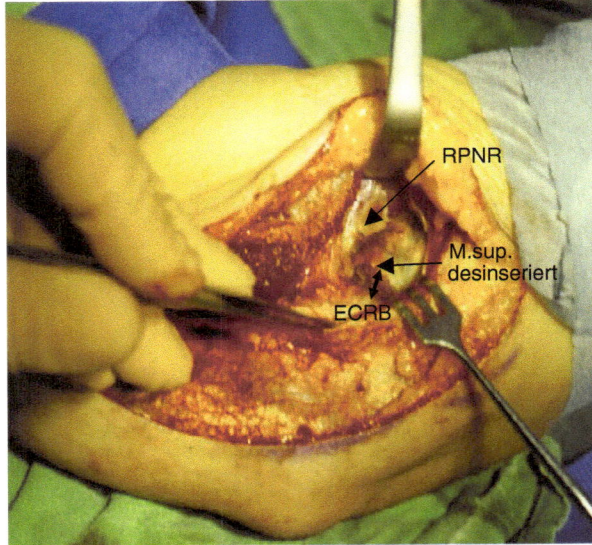

RPNR

M.sup. desinseriert

ECRB

1.8.3 Postoperative Treatment

- Elevation of the arm without inner rotation
- Active motion treatment of fingers and shoulder
- Analgetic and anti-inflammatory treatment
- Removal of drain after 1–2 days

Fig. 1.20 After positioning of Redon drainage into the anterior wound area, all loosened muscle sections are reinserted by continuous absorbable fascia suture 3-4/0, with exception of supinator muscle. (From Wilhelm (2000), with kind permission of Urban and Vogel)

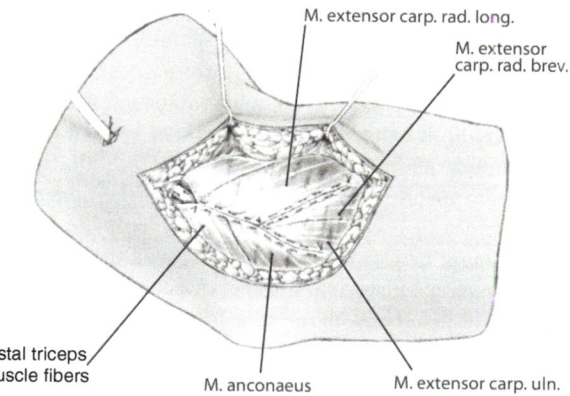

M. extensor carp. rad. long.

M. extensor carp. rad. brev.

Distal triceps muscle fibers

M. anconaeus

M. extensor carp. uln.

- First change of dressing after receding of edema after 1 week
- Removal of skin sutures after 10 days
- Afterwards start of active motion exercise in the elbow joint
- No earlier change of dressing recommendable, as the risk of postoperative swelling or bleeding with lengthening of postoperative course has to be taken into account

1.9   Results

Strictly following guidelines for indication, the *chosen denervation method* with indirect decompression of the deep branch of the radial nerve shows excellent and good results in approximately 93 % (c. Table 1.9, group C II). The remaining 7 % show a fair result, which is positive, as well. Further remarks cf. 1.4, 21–23.

Reviewing literature, already in 1982, the authors of the first publication on denervation by Wilhelm *and* Gieseler (1962) *were attributed the proposal of an extension of the Hohmann procedure and an additional cutting of the posterior cutaneous nerve of the forearm* (Demmer and Rettig 1982). *This is not correct.*

Our publication only elaborates that "by epifascial preparation of the ventral subcutaneous flap the pain conducting branch of the posterior antebrachii cutaneous nerve is already cut" (Wilhelm and Gieseler 1962). Also an extension of the Hohmann procedure is not mentioned. Later publications again and again mention pain, leading fibres of this cutaneous nerve are epifascially cut blindly and unconsciously. There was never the suggestion to prepare the entire cutaneous nerve prior to incision, as stated by Weigel and Nerlich (2005). In addition it has to be mentioned after epifascial blind cutting of the nerve end fibres innervating the epicondyle and the originating portion of the ECRB, there have never been painful small neuromas, contrary to unconsciously damaging the main nerve strand and its branches (Delon et al. 2004).

As a recent development the complete denervation with indirect decompression of the deep radial branch as we recommend since 1991, in literature, is limited to two pain leading strands, the "posterior antebrachii cutaneous nerve and the muscular nerve branch of the anconeus muscle" (Weigel and Nehrlich 2005), not being involved in the main cause of overexertion but only being responsible of the supraepicondyle and posterior pain area innervation.

In the meantime some authors limit the denervation "according to Wilhelm" to only cutting off one nerve, being the collateral lateral branch of the radial nerve. This single neurotomy has already been described by Tavernier in 1946 and today only deserves historical interest due to lack of success. It is performed, however, in complete denervation, in order to extinguish the supraepicondyle pain area.

- *In the interest of the patient, it is advisable to choose the method of denervation successfully used since 1991 and published several times since then.*

This negative situation of publications is worsened by the fact that it obviously does not even seem necessary to anatomically name the nerve that should be cut, only mentioning that "the pain leading nerve runs in the intermuscular bundle of vessels and is cut there".

Lack of information was compensated for by Eisenschenk and Lautenbach (2003) with objective and striking presentation of denervation in the same book, being supported by my own results.

The main danger in surgical procedures in the lateral elbow region *consists of posterior cutaneous antebrachii nerve lesion in anterior incision.* A lesion of the deep branch of the radial nerve can be prevented if division of both radial extensors and incision of the anterior and lateral parts of supinator muscle origin *are performed in pronation of the forearm.*

1.10   Mistakes, Dangers and Complications

- *In contrast to denervation with direct decompression of the deep radial branch, changes of the nerve sliding bed can only be prevented by indirect decompression of the radial nerve, as shown by differing results of both surgical methods* (Table 1.8).

Remaining postoperative complaints can be caused by further proximal irritations of the radial nerve and its references. There is an attempt at conservative treatment after having analysed its localisation.

Pain in the shoulder region is also treated conservatively. Optimised position of the arm in abduction preventing inner rotation is essential.

Swelling of soft tissue and bleeding occur in early removal of Redon drainage and change of dressing. These complications can only be prevented by removing drainage after wound secretions stop and change dressing only after the end of edema. In infection, revision of wound in upper arm discontinuation of blood supply without compression of the arm, drainage, loose wound closure by prepared sutures, immobilisation and antibiotic treatment are necessary. Treatment of rare postoperative Sudeck's dystrophy is discussed in Chap. 5.

References

Almquist EE, Necking WA, Bach AW (1998) Epicondylar resection with anconeus muscle transfer for chronic lateral epicondylitis. J Hand Surg 23A:723–731

van der Beken A, Joveneau B (1983) Traitement chirurgical dú tennis elbow [Surgical treatment of tennis elbow]. Acta Orthop Belg 49:161–183

Bernhart M (1896) Über eine wenig bekannte Form der Beschäftigungsneuralgie [Concerning a rare form of occupational neuralgia]. Neurol Zbl 15:13–16

Bosworth DM (1955) The role of the articular ligament in tennis elbow. J Bone Joint Surg 37A:527–533

Boyd HB, McLeod AC (1973) Tennis elbow. J Bone Joint Surg 55A:1183–1187

Braus H, Elze C (eds) Anatomie des Menschen [Human anatomy], Band 3, 2. Aufl. Springer, Berlin/Göttingen/New York, pp S182–S184, 324–325, 336–337

Buchbinder R, Green SE, Youd JM, Assendelft WJ, Barnsley L, Schmidt N (2005) Shock wave therapy for lateral elbow pain. Cochrane Database Syst Rev (4):CD003524

Capener N (1966) The vulnerability of the posterior interosseous nerve of the forearm. J Bone Joint Surg 48B:770–773

Cohen MS, Romeo AA (2009) Open and arthroscopic management of lateral epicondylitis in the athlete. Hand Clin 25:331–338

Dellon AL, Kin J, Ducic I (2004) Painful neuroma of the posterior cutaneous nerve of the forearm after surgery for lateral humeral epicondylitis. J Hand Surg 29A:387–390

Demmer PJ, Rettig H (1982) Epikondylitis humeri radialis und ulnaris. In: Witt AN, Rettig H, Schlegel KF (eds) Orthopädie in Praxis und Klinik, Bd XI, Teil 2. Thieme, Stuttgart, pp S6.7–S6.30

Dunkow PD, Jatti M, Muddu BN (2004) A comparison of open and percutaneous techniques in the surgical treatment of tennis elbow. J Bone Joint Surg 83B:701–704

Eisenschenk A, Lautenbach M (2003) Nervenkompressionssyndrome [Nerve compression syndromes]. In: Martini AK (ed) Orthopädie und orthopädische Chirurgie. Thieme, Stuttgart, pp S325–S328

Faro F, Wolf JM (2007) Lateral epicondylitis: review and current concepts. J Hand Surg 32B:1271–1279

Fischer AW (1923) Über die Epicondylitis - Styloiditis - Neuralgie, Ihre Pathogenese und zweckmäßige Therapie. [Concerning Tennis Elbow - Styloiditis - Neuralgia, its Pathogenesis and adequate Therapy]. Langenbecks Arch Klin Chir 125:747–775

Frank F (1910) Über die Epicondylitis [Concerning Tennis Elbow]. Dtsch Med Wochenschr 6–13

Garden RS (1961) Tennis elbow. J Bone Joint Surg 43B:100–106

Gardner RC (1970) Tennis elbow: diagnosis, pathology and treatment. Clin Orthop 72:248–253

Goguin JP, Rush F (2003) Lateral epicondylitis. What is it really? Curr Orthop 17:386–389

Goldie I (1964) Epicondylitis lat. hum. (Epicondylalgia or tennis elbow). Acta Chir Scand Suppl 339:1–119

Henry AK (1973) Extensile exposúre. Churchill Livingstone, Edinburgh, pp S113–S119

Heyse-Moore GH (1984) Resistant tennis elbow. J Hand Surg 9E:64–66

Hohmann G (1927) Über den Tennisellenbogen [Concerning tennis elbow]. Verhandlungen der Deutschen Orthopädischen Gesellschaft 21:349–354

Hohmann G (1933) Wesen und Behandlung des sog. Tennisellenbogens [Nature and treatment of so- called tennis elbow]. Münch Med Wschr 7:250–253

Hohmann G (1949) Hand und Arm [Hand and arm]. Bergmann, München

Ishii S, Nakashita K (1985) Entrapment neuropathy of the radial nerve at the elbow – Lateral Elbow pain and posterior interosseous nerve entrapment. In: Kashiwagi D (ed) Elbow joint. Elsevier Science, pp S119–S123

Jalovaara P, Lindholm RV (1989) Decompression of the posterior interosseous nerve for tennis elbow. Arch Orthop Trauma Surg 108:243–245

Kaplan W (1959) Treatment of tennis elbow (epicondylitis) by denervation. J Bone Joint Surg 41A:147–151

Kay NRM (2003) Litigant's epicondylitis. J Hand Surg 28B:460–464

Kupfer DM, Ronson J, Lee GW, Beck J, Gillet J (1998) Differential latency testing: a more sensitive test for radial tunnel syndrome. J Hand Surg 23A:859–864

Lanz T von, Wachsmuth W (1959) Praktische Anatomie [Practical anatomy], 1. Band/3. Teil: Arm. 2. Aufl. Springer, Berlin/Heidelberg

Lishman WA, Russell WR (1961) The brachial neuropathies. Lancet 6:941–947

Major HP (1883) Lawn-tennis elbow. Br Med J 2:557

Morris H (1882) The riders sprain. Lancet 2:133

Narakas A (1987) Allongement proximal du 2 éme radial et neurolyse du nerf radial dans les epicondylalgies rebelles. Swiss Med 7A: 50

Narakas AO, Bonnard C (1993) Epicondylalgia: conservative and surgical treatment. In: Tubiana R (ed) The hand, vol 4. Saunders, Philadelphia, pp S833–S857

Nemoto K, Matsumoto N, Tazaki K, Horiuchi Y, Uchinishi K, Mori Y (1987) An experimental study of the "double crash" hypothesis. J Hand Surg 12A:552–559

Nirschl RP (1994) Tennis elbow: the surgical treatment of lateral epicondylitis. J Bone Joint Surg 61A:832–839

Nirschl RP, Petrone FA (1979) Tennis elbow. The surgical treatment of lateral epicondylitis. J Bone Joint Surg 61A:832–839

Rayan GM, Coray SA (2001) V– slide of the common extensor origin for lateral elbow tendonopathy. J Hand Surg 26A:1138–1145

Reischauer F (1957) Epikondylitis und Tendinitis des Arms, eine Krankheit durch Überbeanspruchung? [Epicondylitis and tendinitis of the arm, a disease by overexertion ?]. Mschr Unfallheilkd 60:321–330

Rineer CA, Rush DS (2009) Elbow tendinopathy and tendon ruptures: epicondylitis, biceps- and triceps ruptures. J Hand Surg 34A:566–576

Roles NC, Maudsley RH (1972) Radial tunnel syndrome. Resistant tennis elbow as a nerve entrapment. J Bone Joint Surg 54B:499–509

Rompe JT, Hopf C, Küllmer K (1996) Extrakorporale Stoßwellentherapie der Epikondylitis humeri radialis – ein alternatives Behandlungskonzept [Extracorporal shock wave lithotripsy of radial epicondylitis – an alternative concept of treatment]. Z Orthop Ihre Grenzgebiete 134:63–66

Runge F (1873) Zur Genese und Behandlung des Schreibkrampfes [Concerning development and treatment of writing cramp]. Berliner Klin Wschr 10:245–248

Rydevik B, Lundborg G (1977) Permeability of intraneural microvessels and perineurium following acute, graded experimental nerve compression. Scand J Plast Reconstr Surg 11:179–187

Schiltenwolf M (2003) Insertionstendinosen – Epikondylitis und Styloiditis [Insertion- tendinosis –Epicondylitis and Styloiditis]. In: Martini AK, Wirth CJ, Zichner L (eds) Orthopädie und orthopädische Chirurgie. Thieme, Stuttgart, p S430

Schmidt HM, Lanz U (1992) Chirurgische Anatomie der Hand [Surgical anatomy of the hand]. Hippokrates, Stuttgart, pp S78–S80

Schneider H, Corradini V (1954) Aufbrauchveränderungen in sehr beanspruchten Sehnen der oberen Extremität und ihre klinische Bedeutung [Overexertion of stressed tendons of the upper extremity and their clinical significance]. Z Orthop u Grenzgebiete 84:278–296

Tavernier L (1946) Epicondylite tenace guéirie par dénervation sensitive régionale. Revue dé Orthopédie 32:61–62

Theis C, Herber S, Meurer A, Lehr HA, Rompe JD (2004) Evidenz-basierte Überprüfung der Therapieempfehlungen bei Epikondylopathia humeri lateralis (Tennisellenbogen) – Eine Übersicht [Evidence- based analysis of suggestions for therapy in lateral epicondylopathy of the humerus]. Zentralbl Chir 129:252–260

Upton ARM, McComas AJ (1973) The double crash in nerve entrapment syndromes. Lancet 2:359–362

Wachsmuth W, Wilhelm A (1967) Zur Ätiologie, Diagnose und Behandlung unklarer Schmerzzustände an der Handwurzel [Concerning etiology, diagnosis, and treatment of obscure pain symptoms at the wrist]. Mschr Unfallheilk 10:89–110

Werner CO (1979) Lateral elbow pain and posterior interosseous nerve entrapment. Acta Orthop Scand Suppl 174:1–62

Weigel B, Nehrlich M (eds) (2005) Operative Therapie der Epikondylitis humeri radialis [Surgical treatment of radial humeral epicondylitis]. In: Praxisbuch Unfallchirurgie, Bd 1. Springer, Berlin/Heidelberg

Wilhelm A (1958) Die Innervation der Gelenke der oberen Extremität [Joint innervation of the upper extremity]. Z Anat Entwckl Gesch 120:331–371

Wilhelm A (1962) Die Innervation des radialen Oberarm-Epikondylen-Gebietes und ihre klinische Bedeutung [Innervation of radial upper arm epicondyle area and its clinical significance]. Z Anat Entwckl Gesch 123:115–120

Wilhelm A (1970a) Das Radialisirritationssyndrom [The radial irritation syndrome]. Handchir 2:139–142

Wilhelm A (1970b) Neues über Druckschäden des N. ulnaris und N. radialis [News on pressure damage of ulnar and radial nerve]. Handchir 2:143–146

Wilhelm A (1972) Die Eingriffe der Schmerzausschaltung durch Denervierung [Surgery for elimination of pain by denervation]. In: Wachsmuth W, Wilhelm A (eds) Die Operationen an der Hand. In: Zenker R, Heberer G, Hegemann G (eds) Allgemeine und spezielle Operationslehre. Band X, Teil III., Springer, Berlin/Heidelberg, pp S264–S285

Wilhelm A (1977) Die Behandlung der Epikondylitis durch Dekompression des N. radialis [Treatment of epicondylitis by decompression of radial nerve]. Handchirurgie 9:185–186

Wilhelm A (1986) Nervenkompressionssyndrome der oberen Extremität unter besonderer Berücksichtigung der Zugangswege. In: Buck-Gramcko D, Nigst H (eds) Bibliothek für Handchirurgie: Nervenkompressionssyndrome der oberen Extremität. Hippokrates, Stuttgart, pp S43–S63

Wilhelm A (1989) Therapieresistente Epikondylitis humeri radialis und Denervationsoperation [Therapy resistant radial humeral epicondylitis and surgery for denervation]. Operat Orthop Traumatol 1:25–34

Wilhelm A (1993) The proximal radial nerve compression syndrome. In: Tubiana R (ed) The hand, vol 4. Saunders, Philadelphia, pp S390–S399

Wilhelm A (1996) Tennis elbow: treatment of resistant cases by denervation. J Hand Surg 21B:523–533

Wilhelm A (1999) Die Behandlung der therapieresistenten Epikondylitis lateralis humeri durch Denervation. Zur Pathogenese [Therapy of resistant lateral humeral epicondylitis by denervation]. Handchir Mikrochir Plast Chir 31:291–302

Wilhelm A (2000) Die Denervation zur Behandlung der therapieresistenten Epikondylitis humeri radialis [Denervation for treatment of therapy resistant radial humeral epicondylitis]. Oper Orthop Traumatol 12:95–108

Wilhelm A (2004) Vortrag: Die Pathogenese des Tennisellenbogens – Konsequenzen für die operative Behandlung [Pathogenesis of tennis elbow - consequences for surgical treatment]. Handchir Mikrochir Plast Chir 36: Abstrakt A 15

Wilhelm A, Gieseler H (1962) Die Behandlung der Epikondylitis humeri radialis durch Denervation [Treatment of radial humeral epicondylitis by denervation]. Chirurg 33:118–122

Wilhelm A, Wilhelm F (1985) Das Thoracic outlet-Syndrom und seine Bedeutung für die Chirurgie der Hand (Zur Ätiologie und Pathogenese der Epikondylitis, Tendovaginitis, Medianuskompression und trophischen Störungen [The throracic- outlet- syndrome and ist significance for hand surgery (concerning etiology and pathogenesis of epicondylitis, tendovaginitis, median compression, and trophic disturbances)]. Handchir Mikrochir Plast Chir 17:173–187

Winckworth CE (1883) Lawn tennis elbow. Br Med J 2:708

The Controversial Pain Syndrome of GE: Pathogenesis and Surgical Treatment of Resistant Cases

2

Contents

2.1 Introduction 33
2.2 Surgically Relevant Anatomy and Physiology 34
2.3 Epidemiology 36
2.4 Aetiology and Pathogenesis 36
2.5 Diagnostics 44
2.6 Classification 46
2.7 Indications and Contraindications 46
2.8 Therapy 46
    2.8.1 Conservative Treatment of GE 46
    2.8.2 Surgical Treatment of GE: Denervation and Circumcision of the Medial
        Epicondyle Region, Area According to Wilhelm 47
    2.8.3 Surgical Treatment of Resistant Cases by Denervation and Subcutaneous
        Transposition of Ulnar Nerve According to Wilhelm 49
    2.8.4 Surgical Treatment by Additional Decompression of the Median Nerve at
        the Cubital Fossa According to Wilhelm 51
2.9 Results 55
2.10 Mistakes, Dangers and Complications 56
References 56

2.1 Introduction

Literature research was accomplished in 1962 as far as it was possible at that time. It was found until then obviously no relevant surgical procedure for the treatment of therapy-resistant "Epicondylitis humeri medialis" had been published. Hohmann in 1949 mentioned this localisation in the context of tennis elbow, especially in diagnostic aspect; he does not describe any relevant surgical procedure, however. In volume 10, part 1 of the *Allgemeine und Spezielle Chirurgische Operationslehre*, a corresponding presentation is missing as well (Wachsmuth 1956).

A. Wilhelm, *Controversial Pain Syndromes of the Arm*,
DOI 10.1007/978-3-642-54513-9_2, © Springer-Verlag Berlin Heidelberg 2015

This fact surprises at first, but it becomes understandable taking into account how rarely golf elbow occurs. Thus, it was advisable to apply the principle of denervation also to the treatment of resistant golf elbow (GE), based on the already promising surgical results in tennis elbow (Wilhelm and Gieseler 1963).

2.2   Surgically Relevant Anatomy and Physiology

Golf elbow (GE), also called thrower elbow (Demmer and Rettig 1982), as a contrast to tennis elbow (TE) only causes slight functional impairment of the hand and is also characterised by a relatively small pain area. This is frequently limited to the peak and the entire circumference of the medial epicondyle. In severe cases also pain areas at the medial collateral ligament and the humeral forearm flexor region of origin, especially the pronator teres muscle, are found. Contrary to TE, where the pain region is solely innervated by fibres of the radial nerve, innervation of the corresponding region in GE is accomplished by branches arising from two main nerve stems, being the median nerve (C7–Th1) and the ulnar nerve (C6–Th1).

The innervation of the medial epicondyle region has already been extensively described by Wilhelm in 1958, 1963 and 1972. *The innervation of the anterior pain area* is mainly accomplished by the final median nerve fibres shown in Fig. 2.1 (right). These arise from recurrent muscle branches, innervating both portions of pronator teres muscle origin as well as of the flexor digitorum communis muscle. The pain-leading fibres can be seen up to the epicondyle peak and the medial collateral ligament. The cranial circumference of the medial epicondyle is innervated by a short branch, arising from both the median nerve and the musculocutaneous nerve. This branch innervates the periosteum below the distal fibres of the brachial muscle coming from the medial intermuscular septum. The peak of the medial epicondyle on the front side is additionally innervated by a delicate branch of a cutaneous nerve, the macroscopic innervation area of which is set off by a hatched area in Fig. 2.1 (right). This is a thin branch of 3 cm length escaping from the posterior branch of the cutaneous medial nerve of the forearm above the epicondyle and then separating dichotomically. The stronger branch runs subcutaneously towards the epicondyle peak separating in a bundle and innervating the anterior proximal area of the epicondyle peak. Shortly afterwards a stronger nerve strand separates, ending together with a little branch of the medial collateral artery above the epicondyle (Fig. 2.2).

The posterior pain area of GE is exclusively innervated by articular and periosteum branches of the ulnar nerve (Fig. 2.1 left). According to Rüdinger (1857), three branches are possible. The upper joint nerve can have diverse strengths and already springs from the main stem several centimetres above the epicondyle, then reaching the anteromedial area of the triceps muscle medial head. Here it can already give a fine thread innervating the humeral capsule above the olecranon fossa. Afterwards the first articular branch is found slightly in front of the triceps muscle tendon with branches in the proximal section of the capsule, medial of the elbow. Figure 2.1 (left) as a variety shows a connection between the first and second articular nerve, together innervating the capsule area. The medial articular nerve usually is stronger

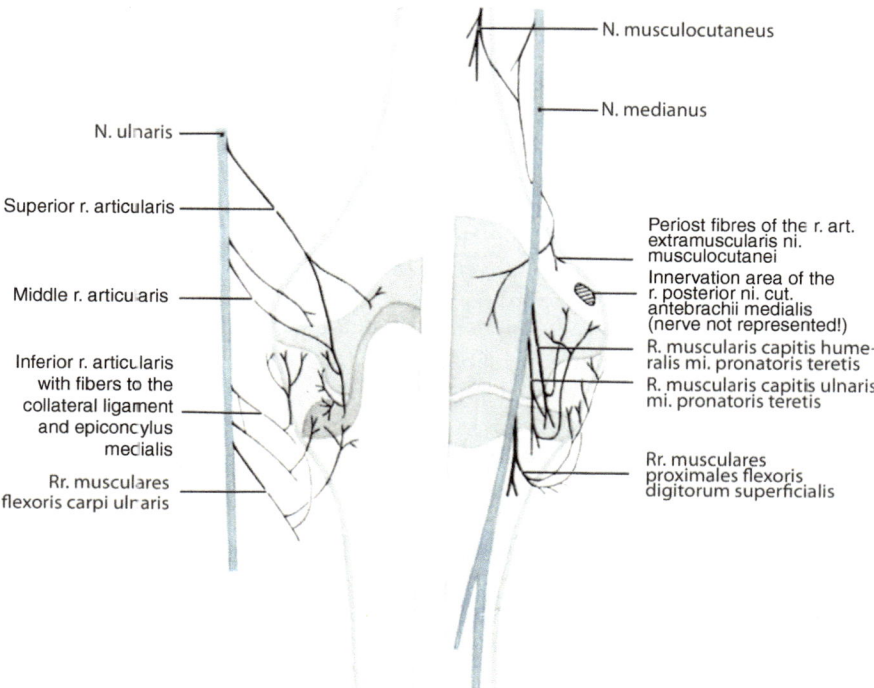

N. musculocutaneus

N. medianus

N. ulnaris

Superior r. articularis

Periost fibres of the r. art. extramuscularis ni. musculocutanei

Innervation area of the r. posterior ni. cut. antebrachii medialis (nerve not represented!)

Middle r. articularis

R. muscularis capitis hume- ralis mi. pronatoris teretis

R. muscularis capitis ulnaris mi. pronatoris teretis

Inferior r. articularis with fibers to the collateral ligament and epicondylus medialis

Rr. musculares proximales flexoris digitorum superficialis

Rr. musculares flexoris carpi ulnaris

Fig. 2.1   Innervation of medial epicondyle region posterior and anterior, ulnar nerve drawn off. (From Wilhelm 1972)

Fig. 2.2   Preparation of medial epicondyle innervation *2* by a branch of the posterior medial cutaneous nerve of the forearm (*1* and *2*), *3* ulnar nerve, *4* epitrochleoanconeous muscle and *5* tendinous arch of ulnar flexor carpi muscle. (From Wilhelm and Gieseler 1963)

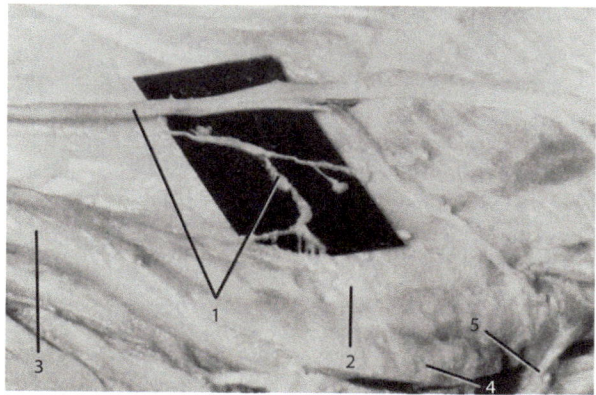

and innervates the distal humeroulnar section of the capsule together with the main branch of the upper articular nerve. A fine fibre, coming directly from the ulnar nerve, might be distinguished between both articular branches, innervating the capsule in the immediate posterior area of the epicondyle massif. The lower articular branch arises either directly from the ulnar nerve or from the proximal ulnar branch, innervating the humeral head of the flexor carpi ulnaris muscle (FCU), with recurrent fibres reaching the collateral medial ligament and the distal medial section of the capsule.

In order to be complete, it has to be mentioned there is a collateral branch of the radial nerve on the medial side as well; it already escapes from the main stem in the axilla and soon afterwards has close connection to the ulnar nerve, breaking through the intermuscular medial septum together in posterior direction and running on the free surface of the triceps muscle medial head in distal direction, finally ending as an articular branch at the olecranon fossa. This branch, however, is not responsible for pain conduction in GE. This is also true for a posterior branch of the medial cutaneous antebrachii nerve, innervating the medial rim of the elbow and the capsular area in the immediate neighbourhood. This is why both nervous branches were not mentioned in Fig. 2.1 (left).

2.3   Epidemiology

Golf elbow (GE) is relatively rare. According to Nigst (1993), its frequency is 5–10 % compared to 90–95 % in tennis elbow. Median age is 43 (21–65) years (Vangsness and Jobe 1991). The authors regarded surgical therapy as necessary in 38 (11.4 %) out of 334 patients. Thirty-five follow-ups consisted of 32 males and 3 females. In 33 out of 35 patients, the symptom affected the dominant arm. Side distribution was 28:7 in favour of the right side. Depending on patient volume, the frequency of GE per year according to Vangsness and Jobe (1991) is 3.5 %; according to Schwarz et al., it is 1.4 %; and in our own patient population, it is 1.1 %.

2.4   Aetiology and Pathogenesis

Anamnestically patients mention occupational as well as leisure activities as exogenous causes of GE, leading to an overexertion of the muscles in the upper arm and the humeroulnar region. In professional life this can be caused either by an acute event, for instance, a sudden sticking fast of a pneumatic drill (so-called backlash injury), or by chronic stress in certain professional procedures, demanding continuous flexion and extension of the elbow joint, especially in combination with simultaneous pronation. A typical example is the ongoing service of the lever of a drill or a punching machine. This exertion can result in pressure damage of the ulnar nerve at its sulcus and the median nerve at the humeral trochlea, possibly also leading to pain radiation in the medial epicondyle region.

Patients with *ulnar nerve irritation* sometimes also report pain in both outer fingers, connected with the sensation of falling asleep and a certain loss of crude strength as well as precision movement. These symptoms are also found in an early proximal ulnar compression syndrome (PUKS), which is not surprising, as identical compression mechanisms cause PUKS and GE.

This also applies to the median nerve. In this case patients complain not only about pain in the cubital fossa and the medial epicondyle region but also about symptoms of an early pronator syndrome. Patients also report a deterioration of pain in the cubital fossa in strong grip. Numbness is minor, but reduction of strength is some stronger.

Still insertional tendopathies and degenerative tendon processes are held responsible as an *endogenous precondition for GE*. Anatomical, clinical and intraoperative findings as a contrast and finally the convincing postoperative results prove that the endogenous precondition in fact is a functionally caused pressure damage of median and ulnar nerve in various extents.

In sports exogenous causes are found in golf, as well as in javelin throw, discus throw, baseball, racketball, bowling, weight lifting, and cross-country skiing (Fulkerson 1980). Weight lifting deserves special interest with regard to pathogenesis. Especially in this discipline, Neugebauer saw (1974, quoted according to Machacek 1976) especially medial "epicondylitis" in 24 weight lifters 19 times altogether.

Promoters of a tendinogenous pathogenesis find a causal relation in pain of golf elbow and insertion tendinopathy or a degenerative process of the muscles coming from the medial epicondyle as result of a functional overexertion (Wirth 2007). The consequence of eliminating the pain by traction relief in shape of a tendon notch or of loosening the originating fibres is convincing at first sight. It was logical then to perform surgery of resistant GE also according to the Hohmann principle (1949). Machacek (1976) among others reported four successfully surgically treated patients, where "the muscle origins were loosened at the medial epicondyle down to the bone". It was not mentioned, however, which muscles were involved.

A similar surgical procedure was also published by Vangsness and Jobe (1991), where after preparation of the epicondyle the common origin of the forearm muscles including the humeral head of the FCU is cut horizontally, loosened, sparing the medial collateral ligament and finally being replaced again. After drilling the epicondyle several times, the loosened forearm flexors are reinserted with several sutures in "length of relaxation" in order to reconstitute the normal muscle tension. Despite this controversial reinsertion, the authors report excellent results in 24 (69 %) out of 34 cases and good results in 10 patients (19 %). This is surprising and cannot be explained from the pathogenetic point of view, as the end of the procedure results in the original traction tension at the medial epicondyle. Again the question arises how pain relief was accomplished in 88 %. A transitory elimination of traction stress at the epicondyle cannot be the reason for the surgical success. If the extension of the corresponding pain area and its nervous supply by final fibres of the median nerve and the ulnar nerve is taken into account, only one explanation remains: *an unconscious denervation*. Here in loosening the anterior soft tissue flap not only the nerve fibres coming from the subcutis to the epicondyle and supraepicondyle are cut but also the pain conducting final fibres of the median nerve muscle branches, providing the supply for the humeroulnar muscles.

The significance of an exclusively neurogenous genesis of GE is supported by the following facts and conclusions:

1. *Anamnestic notes* concerning exogenous causes of GE (cf. above): patients mainly report pain at the inner side of the elbow joint as main symptom, developing or deteriorating in motion of the elbow joint, especially against resistance, for example, in carrying a bag. In maximum extension of the elbow joint, for example, in playing golf and in carrying and lifting heavy weights, pain is reported as well. These pain radiations are also demonstrated by some patients (Fig. 2.15). Additionally minor pain radiation distally and proximally is reported as well as minor disturbance of sensibility and some impairment of crude strength and delicate motion.

2. *Maximum extension of the pain area* does not only include the corresponding epicondyle region but also the humeroulnar muscle origin, being the pronator teres muscle, the flexor digitorum superficialis muscle and the humeral head of the FCU, including the medial collateral ligament.

3. *The anterior pain area* apart from a periosteal fibre of the forearm medial cutaneous nerve posterior branch is mainly innervated by final fibres of median nerve muscular branches destined for the humeral origins of the pronator teres muscle and the superficial finger flexor muscle (Fig. 2.1 right). These structures can be confirmed by a corresponding nerve blockade, at the same time localising the pain area.

4. As early as 1963, "*neuro-irritation impulses*" have been discussed as cause of anterior pain radiation, transferred by the median nerve, the causes remaining obscure, however. Systemic clinical and intraoperative examinations of the median nerve and its proximal myokinetic branches have shown a predominant localisation for irritations in the proximal area of the cubital fossa. This was confirmed in *7 out of 12 surgically treated GE* of this series, supporting that also in GE there are pain radiations caused by further proximal nerve irritation. In the remaining five patients, the cause was finally supposed to be in the area mentioned above.

5. A median nerve and myokinetic branches pressure damage of minor degree (irritation!) at the humeral trochlea, caused by direct *pressure of the bicipital aponeurosis in 5 out of 12 patients* is responsible for the anterior pain radiation (Figs. 2.16 and 2.17). In these cases after resection of the bicipital aponeurosis, a protruding and broadened median nerve with parallel fascicles and missing subepineural blood flow at the humeral trochlea is found in extension of the elbow joint, so also a disturbance of the intraneural flow can be concluded in both remaining cases, clinically initially also presenting as a compression syndrome of the bicipital aponeurosis. The main cause was a pressure damage by a *fascia bridge* of several cm, lying deep and being tense, connecting the pronator teres muscle and the brachial muscle, as well as disturbing the median nerve in its side movement (Figs. 2.18, 2.19, and 2.20). After resection of this fascia, there is a severe disturbance of blood flow and a slight broadening of the nerve diameter and in one case even a circumscribed loosening of the epineurium, as well as a stronger notch. In extension of the elbow joint, the results of this compressing fascial plate are evident (Figs. 2.18, 2.19 and 2.20).

6. As the *bicipital aponeurosis* spreads into the forearm fascia, in contraction of the biceps muscle, a certain functional tension band wiring effect develops, pushing a contracted pronator teres muscle stronger against the humeral trochlea and the brachial muscle above. As a result, also the median nerve and its motoric branches suffer from additional pressure, as shown in two patients. This finding supports the technique of *always resecting the bicipital aponeurosis* in decompression of the median nerve. A neural irritation by a supracondylar process or by a Struther ligament was not seen in this series.

7. *The posterior pain area*, including the origin of the flexor carpi ulnaris humeral head and the medial collateral ligament in contrast to the anterior area, is exclusively innervated by fibres of the *three articular branches of the ulnar nerve* (Rüdinger 1857) (Fig. 2.1 left) and can be extinguished, as well as identified by blocking this nerve 2 cm proximal to the epicondyle peak. On demand, the subcutaneous posterior branch of the cutaneous medial nerve of the forearm can be blocked from here as well. Routine blocks like this are not necessary in GE and TE contrary to wrist denervation.

8. Locally, apart from pressure pain, in some cases limited to the *peak of the epicondyle, an ulnar nerve sensitive to pressure pain in increase of passive flexion radiating pain* in the direction of the epicondyle, sometimes down to the small finger, is found. Slight hypaesthesia can be noticed in this area. Identical symptoms are found in the flexion test of the elbow joint in proximal ulnar compression (PUKS).

9. In pathogenetic aspect of pain radiation to the posterior part, the following *endogenous causes are found as predisposing factors*: in a normal grooved sulcus of the ulnar nerve (Fig. 2.3), the nerve is found dorsal of the elbow joint axis, thus permanently experiencing traction and pressure stress in articular flexion, caused and at the same time caught by the epicondyle mass. Hereby in changing pressure and extension of the joint, the nerve experiences a continuous change of its diameter, resulting in repeated shifting of individual fascicles, change of nerve pressure and traction stress as well as a recurrent medial shift of the nerve. This can even be supported by the effect of the short triceps muscle head. These irritations lead to disturbances of nervous blood flow and axonal flow, basically responsible for pain radiation and the change in surface sensitivity. In a normal epicondyle, there can still be a tendency towards luxation if the ulnar nerve in increasing flexion finds its hypomochlion in the distal area of the epicondyle circumference, at this point moving into a more or less obtuse angle into the trochlea (Güney et al. 1977).

10. Main causes of GE in endogenous aspect are *dysplasia of medial epicondyle and quality of roof* above the ulnar nerve sulcus. Whether there is subluxation or luxation of the ulnar nerve depends on the ulnar nerve sulcus roof stability. This is accomplished either by the *atavistic epitrochleoanconaeus muscle*, first described by Gruber (1866), bridging the sulcus in diagonal direction, innervated by a branch of the ulnar nerve, or by its ligamentary rudiment, being the *epitrochleoanconaeus ligament*. The rudimentary character of this ligament is supported by the fact that it can contain transverse muscle fibres, corresponding

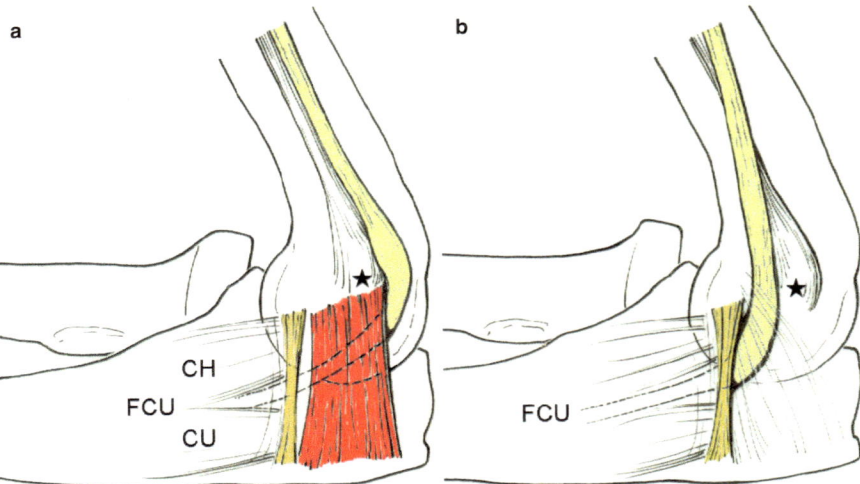

Fig. 2.3 Presentation of ulnar nerve luxation mechanism. (**a**) Proximal compression syndrome in subluxation (Wachsmuth and Wilhelm 1968). (**b**) Distal compression in luxation (Osborne 1957). *Asterisk* medial epicondyle, *yellow* ulnar nerve with pseudoneuroma, *red* epitrochleoanconaeus muscle, *orange* tendinous arch of FCU, *CH* humeral head, *CU* ulnar head. (From Suden and Wilhelm 1987, with kind permission from Thieme)

to the fibre flow of the epitrochleoanconaeus muscle. According to anatomic research, this muscle is found in 17.9–28.7 %, according to clinical findings in 9–17.3 % (Table 2.1). Intraoperatively the muscle was found in 9.0–17.3 % (Table 2.2). The epitrochleoanconaeus muscle and its ligamentary rudiment come from the medial epicondyle mass and connect to the opposite olecranon circumference between articular capsule and final tendon fibres of the triceps muscle medial head (Figs. 2.3 and 2.5). The epitrochleoanconaeus muscle and the ligament develop a rhombic shape in articular extension, whereas in increase of flexion a trapezoid shape develops, due to change of distance and transposition of the points of origin and insertion. At the same time a significant extension of these structures up to one third is accomplished, as seen in Fig. 2.4, leading to a very strong tension of the proximal muscular and ligamentary rim, whereas only a slight lengthening is seen at the distal rim (Fig. 2.6). The epitrochleoanconaeus muscle is innervated by a branch coming from the ulnar nerve together with the upper articular branch (Fig. 2.2) (Wachsmuth and Wilhelm 1968). Mummenthaler (1961) described the tension of the epitrochleoanconaeus ligament, possibly "leading to a compression of the nerve in the sulcus itself"; in this context, the author also elaborates that "the nerve is more or less compressed between the descending triceps and the ulnar epicondyle".

Table 2.1 Epitrochleoanconaeus muscle: anatomic findings

Authors	Preparations	Cases	%
Gruber (1866)	First description		
Kudo a. Li (1956)	472	85	18.0
Mummenthaler (1961)	56	10	17.8
Bando (1979)	157	45	28.7

Table 2.2 Epitrochleoanconaeus muscle: clinical findings

Authors		PUKS	M. epitr.	%
1. James	1956	?	1	–
2. Wachsmuth a. Wilhelm	1968	?	5	–
3. Vanderpool	1968	?	2	–
4. Kojima et al.	1979	44	4	9.0
5. Nigst	1983	338	31	9.3
6. Own patient population	1962–1969	?	16	–
	1970–1984	208	36	17.3

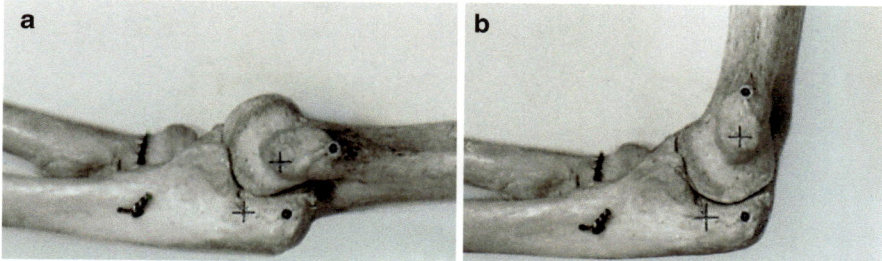

Fig. 2.4 Insertion and origin of epitrochleoanconaeus muscle. (**a**) In elbow joint extension, (**b**) in elbow joint flexion. Distance between the origin and insertion of this muscle and also its ligamentary rudiment increases in continuous flexion and finally leads to a sharp limitation of this structures at the entrance to the ulnar nerve sulcus and their maximum tension

11. In regular presentation, the sulcus and epicondyle shelter the nerve from complete luxation. A tendency towards subluxation is only found in final flexion, being found earlier in epicondyle dysplasia, then resulting in compression of the nerve between the epitrochleoanconaeus muscle in maximum tension or its ligamentary rudiment and the epicondyle peak (Figs. 2.3, 2.4, 2.5 and 2.6). If this position is maintained intraoperatively after loosening the roofing structures, there sometimes is a slight notch of the nerve and scarring of its gliding bed and in all cases a lack of subepineural blood flow as result of compression (Fig. 2.8). James (1956) for the first time reported the possibility of a muscular compressive effect, without demonstrating the pressure mechanism in detail;

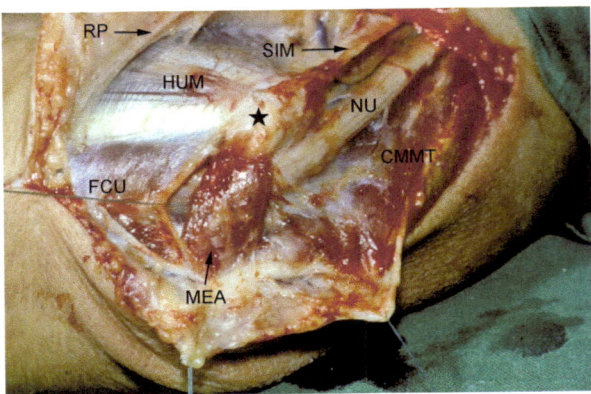

Fig. 2.5 Proximal compression mechanism of the right ulnar nerve if an epitrochleoanconaeus muscle exists. *Asterisk* medial epicondyle, *RP* posterior branch of medial antebrachii cutaneous nerve, *HUM* humeroulnar muscles, *SIM* medial intermuscular septum, *NU* ulnar nerve, *CMMT* triceps muscle medial head, *MEA* epitrochleoanconaeus muscle, *FCU* ulnar carpi flexor muscle; tendinous arch in green suture retracted distally. (From Suden and Wilhelm 1987, with kind permission from Thieme)

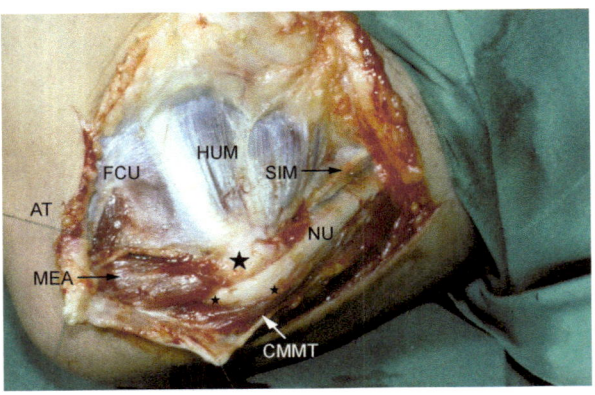

Fig. 2.6 Entrapment of subluxated ulnar nerve between proximal rim of epitrochleoanconaeus muscle and medial epicondyle (*asterisk*). *HUM* humeroulnar muscles, *SIM* medial intermuscular septum, *NU* ulnar nerve, *CMMT* medial head of triceps muscle, area of subepineural disturbance of blood flow in the zone of maximum pressure stress of the ulnar nerve, marked by two *little asterisks, MEA* epitrochleoanconaeus muscle, *AT* tendinous arch of flexor carpi ulnaris muscle. (From Suden and Wilhelm 1987, with kind permission from Thieme)

this is also true for Vanderpool et al. (1968). Only in 1968 the intraoperative proof of this proximal compression mechanism was found in five cases (Wachsmuth and Wilhelm), the results of which can even worsen in ligamentary roofing, as the proximal border of the ligament in maximum tension has the function of an edged structure, even resulting in acute compression damage of the nerve in forced motion, as, for example, in parallel bars.

Table 2.3 Ulnar nerve: luxation mechanism (1970–1984)

$N_{LM} = 131$	$N_{Sublux.} = 77$		$N_{Lux.} = 54$
Mechanism	**Side distribution**		**Frequency**
	Right	**Left**	
A. Subluxation (Suden a. Wilhelm 1987)	38	39	$77 = 58.8\,\%$
B. Luxation (Osborne 1957)	28	26	$54 = 41.2\,\%$
Total	S = 66	S = 65	$S = 131 = 100\,\%$

12. *In missing or insufficient development of the roof above the ulnar nerve sulcus*, the nerve in increase of flexion luxates over the distal section of the medial intermuscular septum and the epicondyle peak frontally and distally. This results in a quasi-rectangular change of course below the tendinous arch of the FCU, maximally flexed in this position, in a relatively tight osteofibrous channel, described as cubital tunnel by Feindel and Stratford (1958). A more or less strong irritation and a trapping of the ulnar nerve at the rim of the anatomically well distinguishable tendinous arch result (Figs. 2.3, 2.10 and 2.11). This can lead to paraesthesia and hypaesthesia in ongoing flexion, for example, during sleep, resolving after extension of the joint. These complaints can be reproduced by flexion test (Wilhelm 1970). In the course of time, this luxation mechanism (Osborne 1957) can lead to remaining sensitive and myokinetic disorders in stress, such as golf elbow and the proximal ulnar nerve compression syndrome. Table 2.3 informs about the frequency of both luxation mechanisms (Figs. 2.3, 2.4, 2.5, 2.6, 2.9, 2.11, 2.12 and 2.13).

13. *GE in so-called double nerve* lesion has a special significance for the pathogenesis. In 100 surgically treated TOS, altogether 23 (23.0 %) GE were found, disappearing after transaxillary decompression of the nerve vessel strand in 19 (82.6 %) out of 23 patients. Only three cases were not influenced.

14. *Similar results in Sudeck's dystrophy* were in 1 (10 %) of 10 cases the clinical picture of GE developed and disappeared after transaxillary surgery.

15. *Checking the trigger test* of the median nerve at the humeral trochlea, there is spreading of pain via pronator teres muscle in the direction of the medial epicondyle (Fig. 2.15).This also occurs in extension test of the elbow joint. A pressure sign was found in 6 out of 7 patients.

16. *A compression of the median nerve by the bicipital aponeurosis at the humeral trochlea*, as already described by Laha et al. in 1978, is found in five cases. After resection of this structure, a protruding and broadened nerve is found in extension with fascicles lying next to another and lack of subepineural blood flow, where a disturbance of the intraneural flow can be concluded as well.

17. Both remaining cases, clinically first also presenting as bicipital aponeurosis compression syndrome, a *fascia bridge of several centimetres, reaching from the pronator teres muscle to the fascia of the brachial muscle*, also hindering the flexibility of the nerve, was found as a possible main cause. After resection of the fascia strip, compression damage was found as a circumscribed detachment of the epineurium and a severe impairment of blood flow. No localisation at the median nerve was clinically found in 5 out of 12 patients.

2.5   Diagnostics

A diligent anamnesis stands at the beginning of examination.

Here pain quality and localisation of pain as well as professional and recreational overexertion of the elbow joint have to be analysed. The motion patterns resulting in stress are important. Sleeping with angled elbows and whether resulting paraesthesia resolves after stretching the arm in outer rotation have to be discussed. Is there pain at the elbow joint moving to the inner side in maximum extension of the arm? Ask for discomfort and numbness of the hand in ongoing flexion (ulnar nerve) and extension of the elbow joint (median nerve).

Concerning the plan of a possible ulnar nerve transposition, it is essential to look for toxic influences (alcohol abuse), metabolic and infectious diseases serving as focal toxics, as the postoperative result, especially in the transposed ulnar nerve, depends on diagnostic clarification and preoperative treatment of these risk factors (Fig. 2.7).

During examination for GE, the possibility of an overlying irritation of median nerve references (C6–Th 1) and the ulnar nerve (C6–TH 1) at the corresponding intervertebral foramina and the thoracic outlet has to be taken into account, as the development of GE is favoured in certain local preconditions in the sense of a *double nerve lesion. Improvement rates* after surgical treatment of TOS are *convincing with 80 %* (Table 4.2).

Also the rare supracondylar process as a possible source of irritation should not be overlooked. Differentiation of TOS from an ulnar nerve irritation at the elbow joint is simple, being confirmed by the proof of sensibility disturbances at the medial cutaneous antebrachii nerve.

Locally the anterior pain area at the origins of the humeroulnar muscles, especially the pronator teres muscle, and afterwards the posterior pain area at the epicondyle and the neighbouring sulcus region are determined. Afterwards the ulnar nerve is examined at the sulcus and the supraepicondyle section in flexion and extension. Pressure sensibility and flexibility of the nerve, its behaviour in flexion in the sense

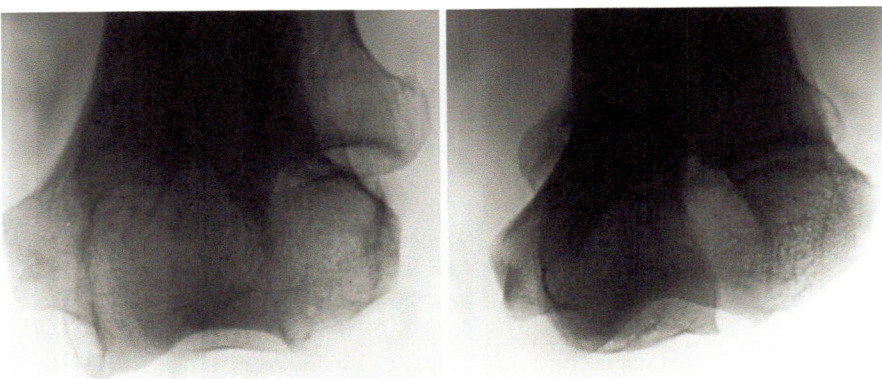

Fig. 2.7 Tangential X-ray of elbow joint in flexion. *Right* normal and *left* dysplastic medial epicondyle. (From Güney et al. 1977)

of a luxation or subluxation, as well as the quality of ulnar nerve sulcus roofing, have to be noticed.

Possibly an epitrochleoanconaeus muscle or its ligamentary rudiment is extremely stretched in maximum flexion and sharply bordered in the proximal area. In subluxation the ulnar nerve is compressed between these structures and the epicondyle peak, and it is sensitive to pressure here. The ulnar nerve behaves in a similar way in luxation based on a lack of roofing above the sulcus, as mentioned before. In this case an entrapment or a compression of the nerve below the tendinous arch of the flexor carpi ulnaris muscle develops, which also hurts at this point. In both cases there is radiation of pain to the posterior area of the epicondyle region; there also is paraesthesia and hypaesthesia, resolving in articular extension. This behaviour of the ulnar nerve is used since 1970 as *flexion test* (Wilhelm) for diagnosis of the proximal ulnar compression syndrome, as well as for GE.

As a contrast, *pain in the anterior area is worsened by palpation of the median nerve trigger points at the humeral trochlea* in arm extension. This provocation of pain can also be accomplished by lifting a chair in an extended arm in supination by increase in pressure strain of the median nerve by the bicipital aponeurosis under tension or possibly by a deep crossing fascia bridge, impairing the median nerve at the trochlea (Fig. 2.19). In this case also peripheral paraesthesia and hypaesthesia can develop in the median nerve area of distribution, disappearing in flexion.

Spinner (cit. according to Tackmann et al. 1989) has noted further manoeuvres for provocation. The compressive effect of the bicipital aponeurosis is evaluated by the pain in forearm flexion and supination against resistance.

Increase in pain in extension of the pronated forearm against resistance supports the compression caused by the pronator teres muscle.

In differential diagnosis the flexion test of the middle finger in supinated forearm against resistance is very important (according to Spinner 1978), as the compressive effect of the superficial tendon arcade on the anterior interosseous nerve (Kiloh-Nevin syndrome) and other neighbouring fibrous anomalies can be either proved or ruled out. In *differential diagnosis* there are foramen stenosis, TOS and traumatic and arthrogenic irritations of the nerve.

X-rays of the elbow joint in two levels to rule out arthrogenic factors and tangential pictures of the ulnar nerve sulcus are recommended for the diagnosis of an epicondyle mass dysplasia (Fig. 2.7).

Neurologic exam of the ulnar nerve in GE is not compulsory if there is a distinct pain area and a positive flexion test. Only in certain cases these exams will be performed due to forensic and differential diagnostic reasons, especially since the localisation of the nerve can be determined exactly by an additional so-called *inching technique*. The ulnar nerve sulcus is covered by an active electrode from distal to proximal direction in 10 mm distance. After passing the area of lesion, there typically is a corresponding jump in latency and amplitude (Kastrup et al. in press).

If the localisation at the median nerve is seen clinically, a neurologic exam should be performed out of differential diagnosis and forensic reasons, also in order to convince the patient of the importance of a second surgical approach with even more reasons.

2.6   Classification

GE is divided into an acute, a resistant to conservative therapy and a chronically recurring form.

2.7   Indications and Contraindications

- *Acute GE primarily needs to be treated conservatively. Resistance to therapy and chronically recurrent disease should be treated surgically but only after having ruled out or having successfully treated a focal toxic process and metabolic disease.*
  Special caution needs to be paid to *alcohol abuse.* Even if it was possible to improve the situation, indication for surgery should only be given after an extensive and forensically clear informed consent, together with a witness.
  In *normal functional behaviour of the ulnar nerve,* simple denervation in shape of a *circumcision of the medial epicondyle region,* where the nerve, prepared in the sulcus, is held by a small Langenbeck or Schiel retractor. In luxation or subluxation of the nerve in GE, a circular denervation with subcutaneous anterior transposition should be performed.
  In *median nerve irritation,* seen clinically and neurologically at the elbow pit, an additional decompression of the nerve has to be performed. Firstly the resection of the bicipital aponeurosis and of deep compressive fibrous structures but also the increase of pressure by the pronator teres muscle on the main nerve stem and its motoric branches have to be seen.
  If median nerve pain clearly dominates pain of the ulnar nerve, possibly after informing the patient and obtaining written consent, the simultaneous procedure at the medial epicondyle does not have to be performed in the medial epicondyle region.
  Elevated infection parameters of obscure cause are a *contraindication.* Also in predominant TOS, surgery for GE should be postponed, taking into account the clear improvement after successfully decompressing the nerve vessel strand according to Roos (1966). This is especially true in Sudeck's dystrophy.

2.8   Therapy

2.8.1   Conservative Treatment of GE

The beginning of conservative treatment in GE is the immediate discontinuation of triggering and entertaining noxae in job and recreation, easily obtained by a transient incapability of working. Immobilising treatment in a well-padded detachable plastic upper arm cast is necessary to prevent extended and repeated flexion of the elbow joint, being placed in flexion of the arm in 0-30-0° in intermediate position of the forearm for 2–3 weeks.

The cast should be worn not only at night but also during daytime, depending on the severity of local findings. Further on during daytime, pronounced flexions of the elbow joint, especially against resistance, have to be prevented, as well as final extension movement under stress, in order to guarantee a pressure relief of the ulnar nerve as well as of the median nerve. *Simultaneous trophic disturbance with hyperhidrosis of the ulnar area possibly needs even longer immobilisation in 0-30°-0 flexion.*

Locally and orally anti-inflammatory therapy is advisable. Prescription of simple painkillers suffices in stronger pain. In very strong pain, an infiltrative anaesthesia at the medial epicondyle can be undertaken.

* *Local injection of corticoid should not be performed.*

At night the arm should be placed high without inner rotation. Shoulder and finger joints can be moved immediately. Discontinuation of immobilisation initially is only allowed during daytime after adequate advice.

2.8.2 Surgical Treatment of GE: Denervation and Circumcision of the Medial Epicondyle Region, Area According to Wilhelm (Fig. 2.9)

2.8.2.1 Informed Patient Consent
* Explanation of possible surgical techniques and information concerning combined procedures, such as transposition of the ulnar nerve, additional decompression of the median nerve in the elbow fossa or revision of a nerve in secondary procedures (relapse), duration of surgery 30–60 min, longer in secondary procedures
* Usual postoperative complaints, like swelling of soft tissue, bleeding and infections
* Remaining complaints, especially in independently persisting areas of disturbance at the upper arm, shoulder, neck and cervical spine
* Possibility of injuring the posterior branch of the medial cutaneous antebrachii nerve, especially in secondary procedures and transient nerve damage by retractor pressure
* Limitation of elbow motion (rare: focal arthritis)
* Sudeck's dystrophy—not found in own patient population
* Cosmetically insufficient scar

2.8.2.2 Instruments
* Hand surgery equipment
* Delicate electric knife

2.8.2.3 Anaesthesia and Positioning
* Intubation anaesthesia, upper or lower plexus anaesthesia and i.v. regional anaesthesia
* Position on the back
* Arm bandage towards the trunk and application of a controlled upper arm partial deprivation of blood supply, cuff pressure 200–300 mmHg
* Positioning of slightly flexed arm in abduction on a tissue padding
* *This procedure as sole measure is only indicated in normal functional behaviour of the ulnar nerve.*

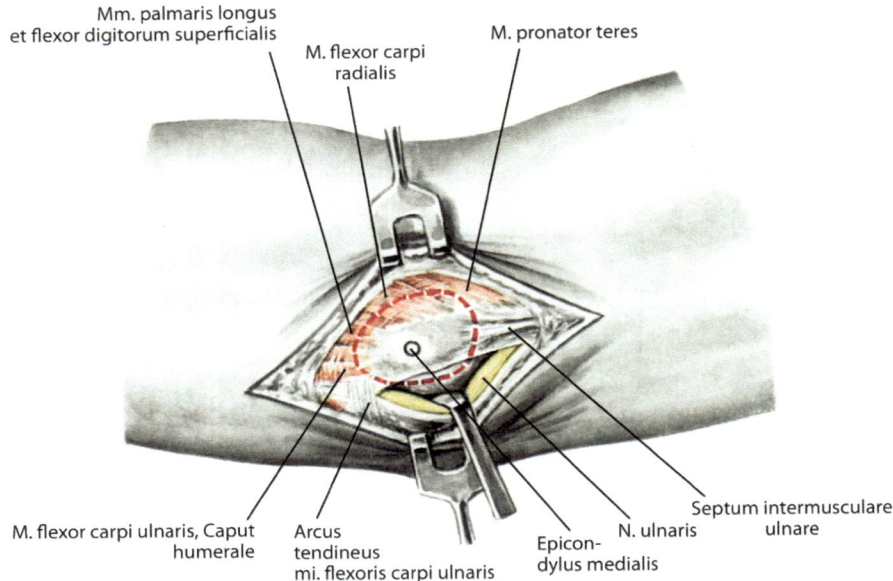

Mm. palmaris longus
et flexor digitorum superficialis

M. flexor carpi
radialis

M. pronator teres

M. flexor carpi ulnaris, Caput
humerale

Arcus
tendineus
mi. flexoris carpi ulnaris

Epicon-
dylus medialis

N. ulnaris

Septum intermusculare
ulnare

Fig. 2.8 Denervation of medial epicondyle region in subluxation missing. *Dotted line* circumcision of the epicondyle, incision of tendinous arch if necessary. (From Wilhelm 1972)

After preparing the surgical site and marking the epicondyle peak, skin is incised in longitudinal direction above the ulnar nerve sulcus in a slight bow shape, starting 3–4 cm proximal and ending distal to the epicondyle peak. Subcutaneous tissue should be prepared with fine scissors in order to take care of the posterior branch of the medial cutaneous antebrachii nerve's variable course. The final fibres of the skin nerve innervating the upper circumference of the epicondyle are cut blindly by epifascial preparation of the soft tissue coat (Fig. 2.1 right). Then the superficial fascia behind the medial intermuscular septum is incised, and the distal roof of the sulcus is cut, diligently sparing the ulnar nerve and its vessels, including the tendinous arch of the FCU, if needed (Fig. 2.8). If there is an epitrochleoanconaeus muscle, it is loosened from the epicondyle in order to open the sulcus. This preparation is necessary to hold the ulnar nerve protected below a retractor during denervation. *A circumcision around the epicondyle* down to the bone suffices for further pain treatment (Figs. 2.1 right and 2.8). A fine electric knife should be used. You start about 1.5 cm above the epicondyle peak and then cut the origin of the humeroulnar muscles in bow shape, including the humeral head of the FCU and the *superficial layer of the medial collateral ligament*, cutting the pain conducting final fibres of the median nerve and the recurrent fibres of the lower ulnar nerve articular branch blindly (Fig. 2.1 left).

Next posterior cutting is performed in 0.5–1 cm from the epicondyle peak, the ulnar nerve being pushed in the direction of the olecranon and remaining under the protection of a small retractor.

After opening the transient deprivation of blood bandage, diligent control of haemorrhage and placing a subcutaneous Redon drainage, the fascial rims including

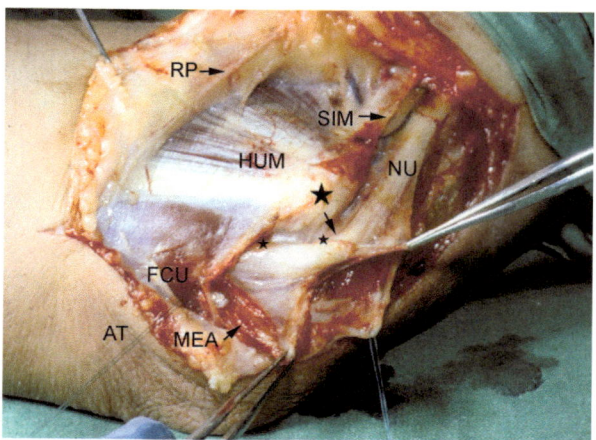

Fig. 2.9 Status post loosening of epitrochleoanconaeus muscle (MEA, *arrow*) from epicondyle after extension of elbow joint. *AT* tendinous arch of ulnar carpi flexor muscle, *asterisk* medial epicondyle, *RP* posterior branch of medial antebrachii cutaneous nerve, *HUM* humeroulnar muscles, *SIM* medial intermuscular septum, *NU* ulnar nerve, *arrow* slight notch and adhesion of paraneural sliding tissue, *small asterisk* ulnar nerve visibly broadened and anaemic, sliding tissue loosened, start of recuperation of subepineural disturbance of blood flow. (From Suden and Wilhelm 1987)

the roof of the sulcus are loosely adapted with resorbable sutures 4–5/0. The wound is closed layerwise, and a compressive dressing is applied reaching from the middle hand to the upper arm. The elbow joint is immobilised in slight flexion (0-30-0) in intermediate position of the forearm and slight extension of the wrist (0-20-0) in an upper arm plastic cast (Figs. 2.8 and 2.9).

2.8.3   Surgical Treatment of Resistant Cases by Denervation and Subcutaneous Transposition of Ulnar Nerve According to Wilhelm (Fig. 2.14)

- *This procedure is only indicated in subluxation and luxation of the nerve, as well as in scarring of its gliding bed.*

It needs a longer bow-shaped incision in order to perform the subcutaneous transpositioning under optimum conditions. The ulnar nerve is prepared as in regular denervation, just a little further proximally and distally in order to obtain a flat run-in run-off angle (Fig. 2.14). The epitrochleoanconaeus muscle or its ligamentary rudiment is detached from the epicondyle (Fig. 2.8) after incision of the superficial fascia, reaching up to the tendinous arch in luxation (Fig. 2.9).

The deep aponeurosis of the FCU is seen after incision of the tendinous arch and separation of both heads of FCU origin, preserving innervation (Fig. 2.13). It is incised longitudinally over a cement spatula and resected in order to prevent a new compression of the ulnar nerve.

Fig. 2.10 Distal compression mechanism of ulnar nerve (*NU*). Ulnar nerve sulcus only covered by superficial fascia. *Asterisk* medial epicondyle, *HUM* humeroulnar muscles, *SIM* medial intermuscular septum, *CMMT* caput triceps muscle medial head, *CUFCU* and *CHFCU* ulnar and humeral head of ulnar flexor carpi muscle; tendinous arch grasped by forceps. (From Suden and Wilhelm 1987, with kind permission from Thieme)

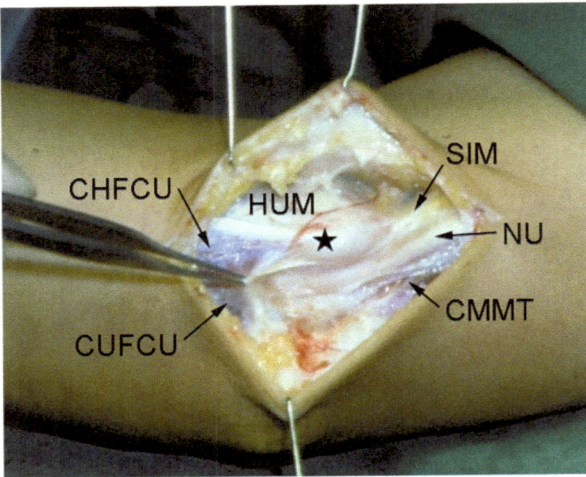

Fig. 2.11 Luxation of ulnar nerve in triceps muscle involvement, entrapment of nerve below tendinous arch marked by spatula. *HUM* humeroulnar muscles, *NU* ulnar nerve, *CMMT* caput triceps muscle medial head, front rim marked by black suture, *AT* tendinous arch, *SIM* medial intermuscular septum, marked by black suture. (From Suden and Wilhelm 1987, with kind permission from Thieme)

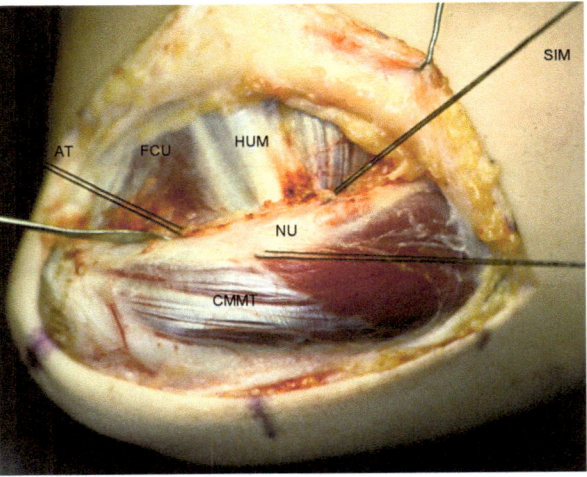

Then the ulnar nerve is cautiously prepared proximally at the septum, snared with a delicate rubber rein and loosened from the sulcus together with its accompanying structures. Joint branches should be cut distally at their innervation site. *Then the distal section of the medial intermuscular septum is resected* in wedge shape, in order to not irritate the transposed nerve (Fig. 2.14). Afterwards there is the typical cut around the epicondyle and diligent control of haemorrhage. After reapplication of the deprivation of blood supply, the anterior wound is checked. In order to limit the extent of the bow-shaped incision, the rims of the wound can be adapted with fine absorbable sutures; only then the transposition of the nerve is performed. In order to prevent relaxation, the nerve has to be retained in its new bed by some absorbable single sutures (4–5/0), connecting the subcutaneous tissue to the superficial fascia at the area of the anterior epicondyle.

Fig. 2.12 Luxation of ulnar nerve and entrapment below tendinous arch (*small asterisks*). *FCU* ulnar flexor carpi muscle, *HUM* humeroulnar muscles, *NU* ulnar nerve; disturbance of blood flow up to the medial epicondyle (*asterisk*). In this position front rim of CMMT reaches medial epicondyle. (From Suden and Wilhelm 1987, with kind permission from Thieme)

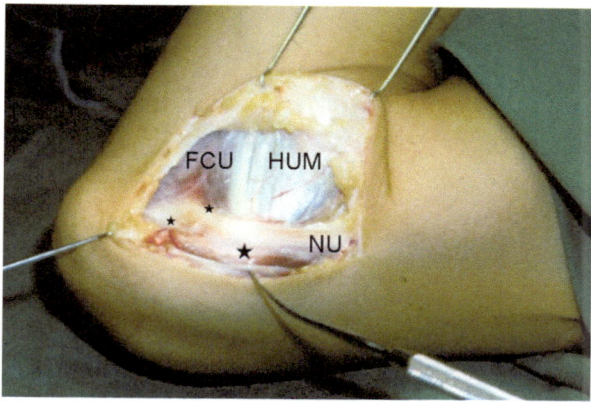

Fig. 2.13 Luxation of ulnar nerve (*NU*) despite elimination of triceps muscle thrust. *AT* cut of tendinous arch marked by black sutures. Deep aponeurosis of flexor carpi ulnaris muscle marked by spatula. (From Suden and Wilhelm 1987, with kind permission from Thieme)

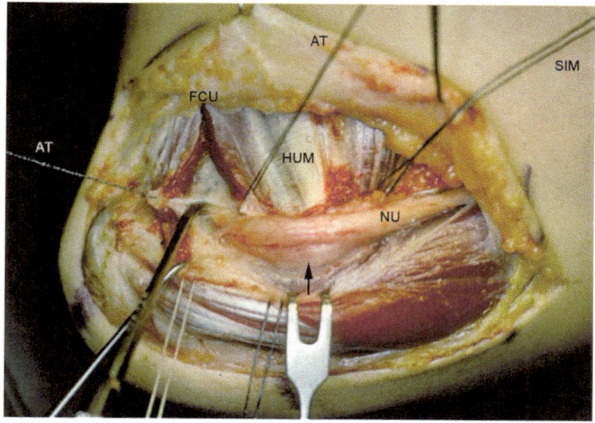

Figures 2.10, 2.11, 2.12 and 2.13 show the ulnar nerve without roof above the ulnar nerve sulcus.

2.8.4 Surgical Treatment by Additional Decompression of the Median Nerve at the Cubital Fossa According to Wilhelm
(Figs. 2.16, 2.17, 2.18, 2.19 and 2.20)

- *In GE this surgical procedure is only performed if irritations of the median nerve at the humeral trochlea are seen clinically and neurologically, responsible for pain radiation into the humeroulnar muscles' area of origin.*

A longitudinal incision suffices for access, starting at the distal upper arm above the medial rim of the biceps muscle, *the medial cutaneous brachii and antebrachii nerves with the basilic vein remaining medial of the incision.* The incision continues directly above the epicondyle line in diagonal direction to the mid of the cubital fossa. This incision can be lengthened in bow shape or zigzag distally, if needed. This

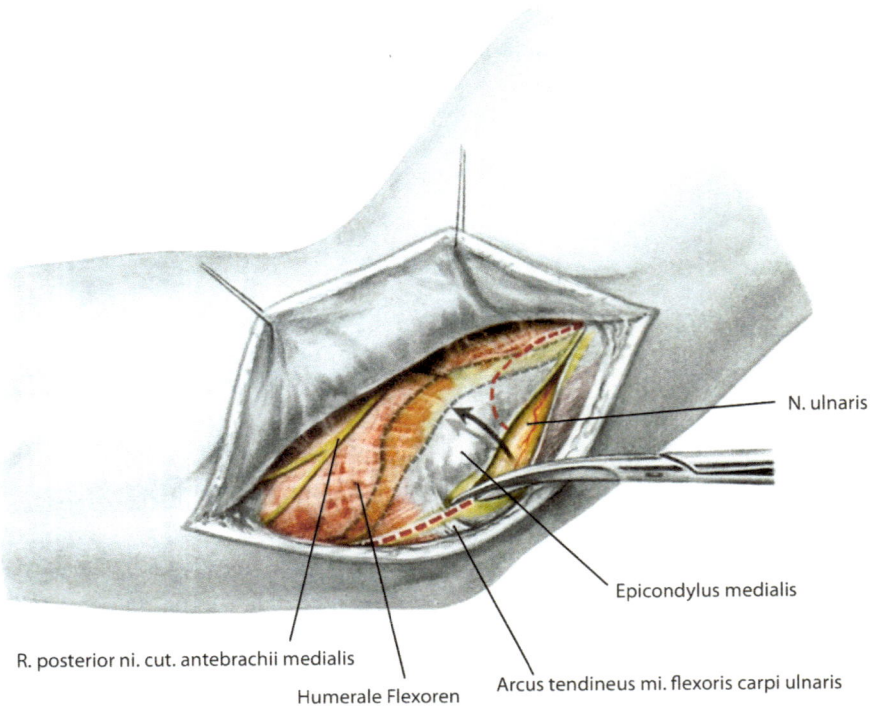

N. ulnaris

Epicondylus medialis

R. posterior ni. cut. antebrachii medialis

Humerale Flexoren

Arcus tendineus mi. flexoris carpi ulnaris

Fig. 2.14 Denervation of medial epicondyle region with subcutaneous transposition of the ulnar nerve in luxation and subluxation. *Red hatched line*, proximal: resection of medial intermuscular septum; *red hatched line* distal: incision of ulnar nerve sulcus roofing, tendinous arch and superficial fascia between both heads of flexor carpi ulnaris muscle origin. (From Wilhelm 1972, Mittelbach 1972)

approach corresponds with the course of the median nerve and the upper rim of the pronator teres muscle. After cutting the superficial fascia follows the resection of the bicipital aponeurosis and the revision of the median nerve to its entry into the pronator teres muscle. The entry of the median nerve below the bow-shaped arcade of FDC can be reached from here. This revision, also including ruling out a supracondylar process and a Struther ligament, is essential, as the nerve can be exposed to diverse irritating and compressing structures at different sites simultaneously, as described by Hartz et al. (1981), Tackmann et al. (1989) and Nigst (1993) (Fig. 2.14).

The median nerve is initially presented at the medial side of the vessel bundle proximal to the bicipital aponeurosis (Figs. 2.15, 2.16 and 2.17). After resection of this structure, connecting the biceps and the pronator teres muscle in shape of a tension strapping, the nerve section with pressure damage is exposed above the humeral trochlea, crossed and padded by the brachial muscle (Fig. 2.17). Then the nerve is revised without lifting it off its gliding bed and observed further distally until the entry into the pronator teres muscle, additionally removing all compressive structures in question. At this point also the myokinetic branches of the median nerve coming from the medial side have to be examined which can mainly be compressed by a hypertrophic pronator teres muscle.

Fig. 2.15 Palpatory examination of median nerve in cubital fossa, marked by small crosses, pain radiation via pronator teres muscle and superficial flexor digitorum muscle in direction of epicondyle region (*arrows*) and in direction of the hand (*blue arrow*) in case of GE. *Asterisk* medial epicondyle

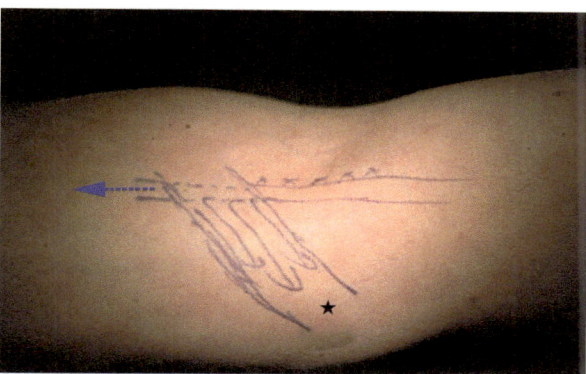

Fig. 2.16 Subfascial site with presentation of bicipital aponeurosis (*LF*) and medial nerve vessel bundle. *AB* brachial artery with accompanying veins, *NM* median nerve, *MPT* pronator teres muscle, *LF* bicipital aponeurosis, *MBB* biceps brachii muscle

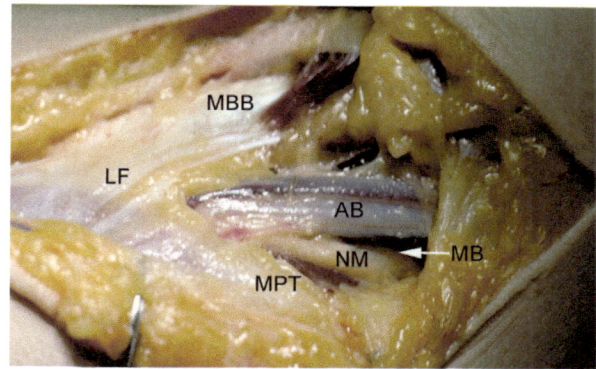

Fig. 2.17 Status post resection of bicipital aponeurosis. In extension of the elbow joint, a protruding and broadened segment (*arrow*) of median nerve (*NM*) with parallel fascicles and absence of subepineural blood flow. *MB* brachial muscle, *PNG* paraneural sliding tissue, loosened, *MPT* pronator teres muscle

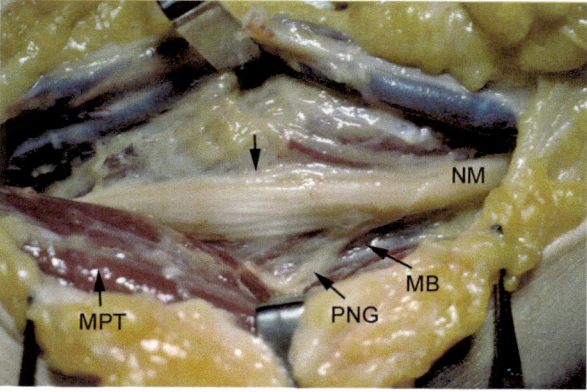

In the depth, proximal of the bicipital aponeurosis, an additional compressive structure is found, a rough fascia bridge crossing the nerve in diagonal direction impairing its motion (Figs. 2.18 and 2.19). The intense compressive effect in this case leads to a massive disturbance of blood flow, well recognisable distal to the structure. After resection of this fibrous bridge, you see the true extent of pressure

Fig. 2.18 Subfascial site in elbow joint extension with presentation of lacertus fibrosus (*LF*). *NM* median nerve, *VB* brachial vessels, *MBB* biceps brachii muscle

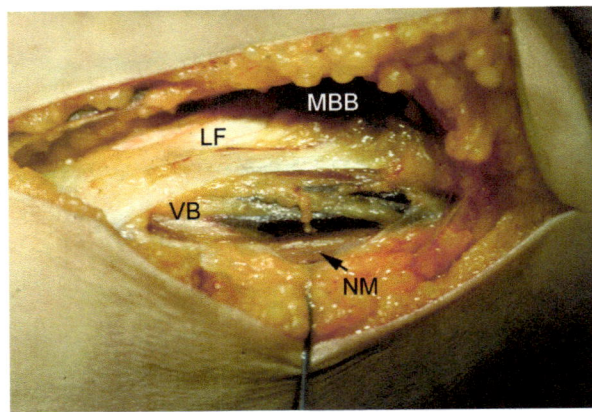

Fig. 2.19 Status post resection of bicipital aponeurosis with presentation of compressing fascia bridge (FB, *arrow*) at the humeral trochlea. Medial nerve with regular blood supply proximally, whereas distal to fascia bridge an anaemic zone is found due to absence of subepineural blood supply. *MB* brachial muscle, *MPT* pronator teres muscle, *VB* brachial vessels, *MBB* biceps brachii muscle

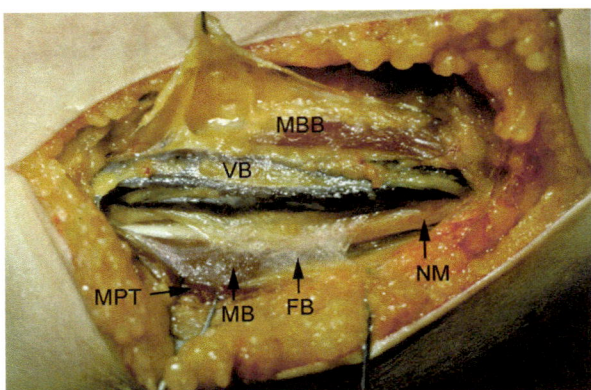

Fig. 2.20 After resection of fascia bridge, a slightly broadened median nerve (*NM*) is found at the site of pressure damage with initial recovery of subepineural blood flow. *MB* brachial muscle, *PNG* paraneural sliding tissue, loosened, *MPT* pronator teres muscle

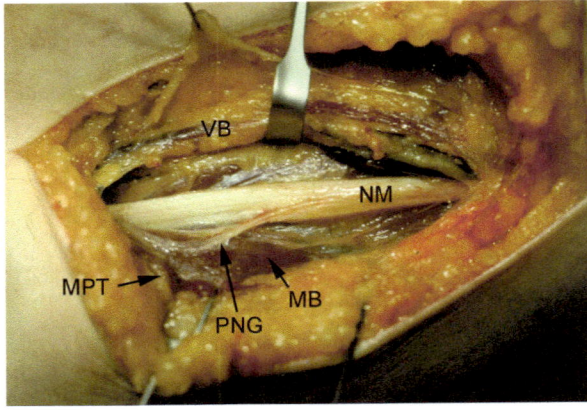

damage (Fig. 2.20), being an extensive disturbance of blood flow and a tangential loosening of paraneural sliding tissue. This kind of pressure damage can also be responsible for pain radiation into the medial epicondyle region. After completing nerve decompression, diligent control of haemorrhage, application of a Redon drainage and closure of the wound layer by layer are necessary (dressing, immobilisation and postoperative care cf. above).

2.9 Results

In our population of 12 patients, clinically and intraoperatively altogether seven distinct pressure damages of the median nerve were found, caused by the bicipital aponeurosis in five cases and caused by a deep fascia bridge in two patients. Only in one out of five patients, sole decompression of the median nerve leads to complete freedom from pain at the epicondyle area and to a reduction of the complaints of the hand (Figs. 2.15, 2.16 and 2.17). In the remaining four patients, the medial denervation had to be performed despite initially little complaints in the ulnar area in a second session. Thus, it has to be concluded both procedures should be undertaken in one session, if possible, if the patient agrees. Otherwise sole decompression of the median nerve should be limited to cases without any symptoms at the ulnar region and a negative flexion test. In seven median decompressions postoperatively, five excellent and one good and one sufficient result each were found.

The median nerve decompression described in the prior section was only performed in one case (result: excellent), whereas the remaining four patients (group B) needed a medial denervation with frontal transposition of the ulnar nerve in a second session (result: excellent and good two times each). The positive result of 91.6 % should not be overrated due to the small patient population.

All pronator symptoms from 1980 to 1994 were checked in order to comment on the frequency of median nerve compression by the bicipital aponeurosis (Laha syndrome) and by a deeper fascia bridge, described by Nigst (1993) as "fibrous sail". A Laha syndrome was found in 9 (40.9 %) out of 22 cases and in 6 (27.3 %) patients compression by a deep fibrous structure, bridging from the brachial muscle to the upper rim of the pronator teres muscle (Laha et al. 1978). One supracondylar process was discovered in this series.

The success rate of surgical treatment mainly depends on the quality of nerve gliding ability after subcutaneous transposition of the ulnar nerve. In adhesions or even scarring of the new gliding bed, the differing traction stress of basal nerve fascicles in extension of the elbow results in complaints essential for the success of surgery. In extreme pain a diligent neurolysis of the ulnar nerve and a repeatet subcutaneous transposition and that under taking care of the posterior cutaneous nerve of the forearm.

Taking into account the mistake of a small patient population, resulting from the rareness of GE, as well as diverse surgical methods, a success rate of 90 % can be expected in this disease. A reduction of excellent results to 58.3 % compared to good results in 33.3 % has to be seen compared to surgical results in TE (Table 1.8, group A, C1 and C2). A fair result was only found in two cases (7.1 %) (evaluation scheme in Table 1.6).

2.10   Mistakes, Dangers and Complications

The deep branch of the medial cutaneous antebrachii nerve can be injured by sharp incision of the subcutaneous tissue. An insufficient deletion of pain is only possible if denervation is not performed lege artis, and a *double nerve lesion* as well as a *focal toxic happening* has been overlooked.

After *decompression of the median nerve,* pain can persist if the distal part of the nerve until its entry into the pronator muscle is not revised. *In any case the bicipital aponeurosis should be resected to reach freedom of pain.*

Surgical revision is indicated in painful adhesion of the transposed ulnar nerve, especially checking the proximal run-in of the nerve at the resected septum and the distal run-off. In a too steep run-off angle after neurolysis, a further division of both FCU origin heads is recommended together with corresponding sharp angled correction of the neural course, being secured by several sutures, fixating the subcutis at the muscular fibres.

Outer neurolysis is needed in scarred bedding of the ulnar nerve, and in severe pressure damage with disturbance of blood flow also a longitudinal epineurotomy without injuring the subepineural vessels is necessary.

An epineurectomy should not be done due to the intense danger of jeopardising the nervous blood supply. Interfascicular neurolysis, as well, should only be considered with extreme caution as the ulnar nerve is rich of sympathetic fibres with the *danger of causalgia.*

If outer neurolysis and epineurotomy do not suffice for solving the pain problem, first the possibility of a *nerve bedding* between outer and deeper vessels and nerve conducting layer of the subcutis should be checked. This method has been valuable in *cheiralgia.*

Swelling of soft tissue and bleeding can only be prevented if the compressive dressing with elastic bandage is applied lege artis, Redon drainage is only removed after secretions stop, and the first change of dressing is only undertaken after the end of the edema phase, that is, only after 1 week. The usual change of dressing on the 1st day after surgery can result in edema with postoperative treatment for 3 months and disability to work.

In infected wound smear, removal of sutures in superficial and revision of wound in deeper process are needed in the upper arm, with partial deprivation of blood supply without bandaging the arm towards the trunk. After application of a Redon drainage of higher calibre, a loose wound closure using the prepared sutures can be used. After application of dressing, immobilisation of the elbow joint and higher positioning of the arm as well as antibiotic treatment follow. A thorough drainage treatment can be necessary in severe infection.

The treatment of postoperative Sudeck's dystrophy is discussed in Chap. 5 (Wilhelm 1997).

References

Bando K (1979) Musculus epitrochleo-anconaeus. Hirosaki Igaku 7:192
Demmer PJ, Rettig H (1982) Werfer-Ellenbogen [Thrower's elbow]. In: Witt AN, Rettig H, Schlegel KF (eds) Orthopädie in Praxis und Klinik, vol XI. Thieme, Stuttgart, pp S6–S18, Teil 2

Feindel W, Stratford J (1958) The role of the cubital-tunnel in tardy ulnar palsy. Can J Surg 1:287–300

Fulkerson JP (1980) Transient ulnar neuropathy from Nordic skiing. Clin Orthop 153:230–231

Güney U, Wilhelm A, Wulle C (1977) Funktionelle Mechanismen des proximalen Ulnariskompressionssyndrom [Functional mechanisms of proximal ulnar compression syndrome]. Handchirurgie 9:193–197

Gruber W (1866) m. Acad. St. Petersburg; VII, S 10, 5

Hartz CR, Linscheid RL, Gramse RR, Daube JR (1981) The pronator teres syndrome: compressive neuropathy of the median nerve. J Bone Joint Surg 63:885–890

Hohmann G (ed) (1949) Hand und Arm – Ihre Erkrankungen und deren Behandlung [Hand and arm - their diseases and treatment]. Bergmann, München, pp S141–S144

James GGH (1956) Nerve lesions about the elbow. J Bone Joint Surg 38B:589

Kastrup et al. (in press) Leitlinien der dtsch. Gesellschaft für Neurologie: Diagnostik und Therapie der chronischen Ulnarisneuropathie am Ellenbogen (ulnar neuropathy at the elbow, UNE) [Guidelines of German Neurologic Society: diagnostics and therapy of chronic ulnar neuropathy at the elbow]

Kojima T, Kurihara K, Nagano T (1979) A study on operative findings and pathogenetic factors in ulnar neuropathy at the elbow. Handchirurgie 11:99–104

Kudo K, Li CN (1956) Concerning frequency of epitrochleoaneous muscle. Hirosoki Med 7:192

Laha RK, Lunsford LD, Dujovny M (1978) Lacertus fibrosus compression of the median nerve. J Neurosurg 48:838–841

Machacek J (1976) Die Hohmann'sche Operation am ulnaren Epicondylus humeri [The Hohmann surgical procedure at the ulnar humeral epicondyle]. Arch Orthop Unfall 85:101–103

Mittelbach HR (1972) Nervendruckschäden [Nerve compression damages]. In: Wachsmuth W, Wilhelm A (eds) Die Operationen an der Hand. Springer, Berlin/Heidelberg, p S255, In: Zenker R, Heberer G, Hegemann G (Hrsg) Allgemeine und Spezielle Operationslehre. Band 10/3

Mummenthaler M (1961) Die Ulnarisparesen [Ulnar Pareses]. Thieme, Stuttgart

Nigst H (1993) Kompressionssyndrome des Nervus medianus im Ellenbogenbereich [Compression syndromes of median nerve at the elbow]. Oper Orthop Traumatol 5:40–47

Osborne GV (1957) The surgical treatment of tardi ulnar neuritis. J Bone Joint Surg 39B:782

Roos DB (1966) Transaxillary approach for first rib resection to relieve thoracic outlet syndrome. Techniques Illustrated. 2:3–13

Rüdinger N (1857) Die Gelenknerven des Menschlichen Körpers [The articular nerves of the human body]. Ferdinand Enke, Erlangen

Spinner M (1978) Injuries to the major branches of peripheral nerves of the forearm, 2nd edn. Saunders, Philadelphia

Suden R, Wilhelm A (1987) Das proximale Ulnariskompressionssyndrom unter besonderer Berücksichtigung des M. epitrochleoanconaeus [The proximal ulnar compression syndrome with special consideration of the epitrochleoanconeous nerve]. Handchirurgie 19:33–42

Tackmann W, Richter HP, Stöhr M (eds) (1989) Kompressionssyndrome peripherer Nerven [Compression syndromes of peripheral nerves]. Springer, Berlin/Heidelberg, pp S144–S151

Vanderpool DW et al (1968) Peripheral compression lesions of the ulnar nerve. J Bone Joint Surg 50B:792–803

Vangsness CT, Jobe FW (1991) Surgical treatment of medial epicondylitis, results in 35 elbows. J Bone Joint Surg 73B:409–411

Wachsmuth W (1956) Die Operationen an den Extremitäten [Surgery of the upper extremity]. In: Guleke N, Zenker R (eds) Allgemeine und spezielle chirurgische Operationslehre, vol X. Springer, Berlin/Heidelberg, p S438, Teil 1

Wachsmuth W, Wilhelm A (1968) Der M. epitrochleoanconaeus und seine klinische Bedeutung [The epitrochleoanconeous nerve and its clinical significance]. Mschr Unfallheilk 71:1–22

Wilhelm A (1958) Zur Innervation der Gelenke der oberen Extremität [Concerning articular innervation of the upper extremity]. Anat Entwickl Gesch 120:331–371

Wilhelm A (1970) Neues über Druckschäden des N. ulnaris und N. radialis [News on pressure damage of the ulnar and the radial nerve]. Handchirurgie 2:143–146

Wilhelm A (1972) Die Eingriffe der Schmerzausschaltung durch Denervation [Surgical procedures for pain elimination by denervation]. In: Wachsmuth W, Wilhelm A (Hrsg) Die Operationen an der Hand. In: Zenker R, Heberer G, Hegemann G (Hrsg): Allgemeine und Spezielle Operationslehre. Band 10/3. Springer, Berlin/Heidelberg, pp S264–S285

Wilhelm A (1997) Operative Behandlung der therapieresistenten Sudeck'schen Dystrophie durch transaxilläre Dekompression des Nervengefäßstranges und Sympathektomie [Surgical treatment of resistant Sudeck's dystrophy by transaxillary decompression of the nerve- vessel- bundle and sympathectomy]. Zur Pathogenese des M. Sudeck. Handchir Mikrochir Plast Chir 29:60–72

Wilhelm A, Gieseler H (1963) Die Behandlung der Epicondylitis humeri ulnaris durch Denervation [Treatment of ulnar humeral epicondylitis by denervation]. Chirurg 34:80–83

Wirth CJ (2007) Degenerative Erkrankungen [Degenerative diseases]. In: Wirth CJ, Mutschler W (eds) Praxis der Orthopädie und Unfallchirurgie. Thieme, Stuttgart/New York, p S867

The Controversial Pain Syndrome of Proximal Radial Compression Syndrome (PRKS): Pathogenesis and Surgical Treatment of Resistant Cases

3

Contents

3.1　Introduction 59
3.2　Surgically Relevant Anatomy and Physiology 61
3.3　Epidemiology 63
3.4　Aetiology and Pathogenesis 63
3.5　Diagnostics 68
3.6　Classification 69
3.7　Therapy 71
　　　3.7.1　Conservative Treatment 71
　　　3.7.2　Surgical Treatment 71
3.8　Results 75
3.9　Mistakes, Dangers and Complications 78
References 80

3.1 Introduction

At the axilla and the upper arm, the radial nerve can be damaged by acute and chronic pressure influence, depending on the strength and duration of the influence even leading to paresis.

Exogenous causes at the axilla may be the incorrect use of crutches, supporting body weight resulting in pressure damage of the nerve between the proximal section of the humerus and the tendons of the latissimus dorsi and teres major muscles (Tackmann et al. 1989). Pressure damage of the radial nerve is more frequent in the course of its flat spiral channel, as here it runs in direct contact with the humeral shaft. Typical examples are the "park paralysis", the "Saturday-night paralysis" and the "Paralysie des Amoureux", which can develop in sleeping deeply, further on the paralysis caused by tourniquet and by position, during surgical procedures with anaesthesia. In literature the special vulnerability of the radial nerve at the spiral channel is connected to its unique situative conditions at the humeral shaft. Further

A. Wilhelm, *Controversial Pain Syndromes of the Arm*,
DOI 10.1007/978-3-642-54513-9_3, © Springer-Verlag Berlin Heidelberg 2015

damage of the radial nerve can occur during birth, by compression, by traction or by masses (haematoma, tumour).

There was no proof of the existence of a proximal radial nerve compression mechanism, even though Gowers as early as 1892 reported three complete radial pareses after a sudden contraction of the triceps muscle, for instance, by throwing a heavy stone. Similar pareses have been described in the past, especially after chronic overexertion of the triceps muscle, as in harbour and garbage workers, weavers,

Table 3.1 Proximal radial compression syndrome (PRKS): N_p (1969–1990) = 30, N_{op} = 30

						Causes		
Pat. no.	Operation no. /year	m	w	Age	Profession	Loc. R/L	Acute trauma	Chron. trauma	Triggering factor
1	1,263/69	+		27	Machine setter	L		+	Ball callus
2	1,560/69	+		63	Metal worker	R		+	Profession
3	2,670/69	+		34	Driver	L		+	Profession
4	2,746/69		+	65	Housewife	R		+	Osteitis
5	238/70	+		27	Drill worker	L	+		Profession
6	785/70	+		41	Varnisher	L		+	Profession
7	1,364/70	+		20	Plumber	L		+	Osteitis
8	1,648/70		+	50	Retired	R		+	Anat. spec. feature
9	3,050/70		+	65	Housewife	L	+		FA-fracture
10	275/71	+		50	Bricklayer	L		+	Profession/anat. spec. feature
11	3,625/71		+	63	Housewife	R		+	Edema/TIS
12	1,721/72	+		45	Worker	R		+	Profession
13	3,096/73		+	40	Housewife	R		+	FA-pseudarthrosis
14	3,339/75	+		26	Roughcaster	R	+		Hard work
15	3,357/75	+		37	Bricklayer	R	+		Hard work
16	1,666/78	+		52	Bricklayer	R		+	Profession
17	1,838/78		+	19	Seamstress	L		+	Profession
18	3,103/78	+		38	Worker	L		+	FA-fracture/AO-PL
19	983/80		+	48	Housewife	L		+	Edema/TIS
20	1,859/84		+	57	Housewife	L		+	Anat. spec. feature
21	1,958/84	+		70	Retired	L		+	Intraneur. splinter
22	2,921/84	+		45	Carpenter	R	+		FA-fracture/AO-PL
23	2,674/86	+		18	Student	R	+		FA-fracture/nail
24	2,796/86		+	46	Hairdresser	R		+	Edema/TIS
25	2,066/87		+	45	Housewife	L		+	Edema/TIS
26	730/88	+		33	Examiner	L	+		FA-fracture/AO-PL
27	1,799/88		+	47	Draftsman	L		+	Anat. spec. feature
28	11.11.89	+		66	Retired	L		+	FA-fracture
29	07.11.90		+	38	Nurse	L		+	Anat. spec. feature
30	13.09.90		+	49	Housewife	L		+	Anat. spec. feature

Seven further patients could not be judged due to loss of data. The complete number of PRKS surgically treated thus amounts to 37

Table 3.2 PRKS
– patient – population:
N_p (1969–1990)=30, N_{op}=30.
Follow-ups: 27[a]+(3[b])

Age	(18–70) Ø 45 years
Sex	17m: 13 f
Localisation (right:left)	12:18
Triggering causes:	
Occupation	11
Upper arm fracture	8 (sec. pareses)
Upper arm osteitis	2
Hand edema (TOS)	4
Intraneural fragment	1
Anatomical variety	4
Radial nerve trauma:	
Acute	7
Chronic	23

[a]Follow-up 1988, published 1993
[b]Follow-up of patients 28, 29 and 30 not possible, as documentation
is missing

waiters and violinists. This is also true for secondary pareses in the further course of
an upper arm fracture and in infectious and tumourous change, already predicting
the existence of a proximal compression mechanism at the upper arm.

Only accidental work with radial paresis after certain motion patterns in the elbow
joint with overexertion of the triceps muscles, for example, after long travels by car,
and in work with compressed air equipment in 1969 led to a solution concerning
localisation and pathogenesis of a proximal radial compression syndrome (PRKS),
first published by Wilhelm in 1970 (Tables 3.1 and 3.2), based on eight patients surgically treated in the Surgical Department of the Teaching Hospital Aschaffenburg
between 1969 and the beginning of 1970.

3.2   Surgically Relevant Anatomy and Physiology

Main areas for this kind of compression are the tendinous portion of origin of the triceps muscle lateral head, crossing the radial nerve directly in front of the lateral intermuscular septum (Fig. 3.2b), and the hiatus of the radial nerve. The latter functions as
a relatively short osteofibrous channel, which can as an exemption also be supplemented by crossing fibrous strands running from the humeral shaft or the base of the
brachial muscle to the septum (Fig. 3.3b).

Bosworth in 1971 already accepted the compression mechanism we described as
explanation for the relatively frequent radial pareses in garbage workers. In the same
year Lotem et al. (1971) confirmed PRKS, based on anatomic examinations and three
patients treated conservatively. They also blamed a fibrous arcade of the lateral head of
the triceps muscle as compressive cause (Bosworth DM, 1971, personal information).

The first surgical confirmation of PRKS was published by Manske (1977).
Further publications are by Lubahn and Lister (1983), Wilhelm and Suden (1985),

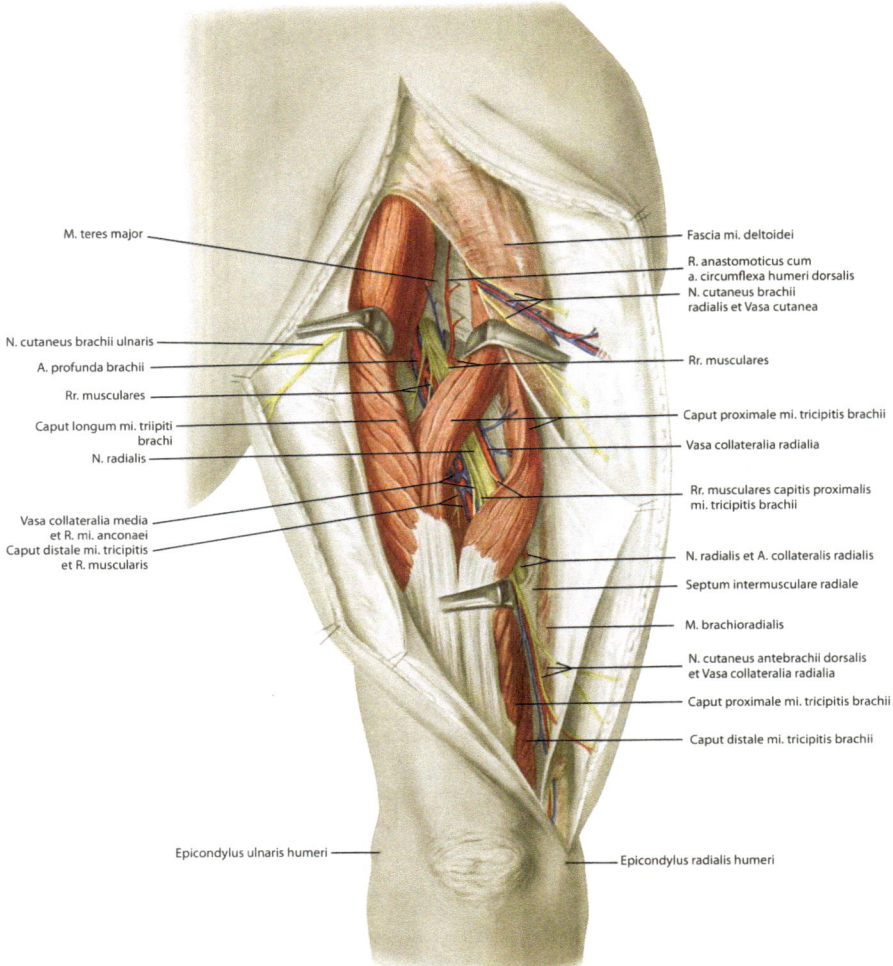

Fascia mi. deltoidei

R. anastomoticus cum
a. circumflexa humeri dorsalis

N. cutaneus brachii
radialis et Vasa cutanea

M. teres major

N. cutaneus brachii ulnaris

A. profunda brachii

Rr. musculares

Rr. musculares

Caput longum mi. triipiti
brachi

Caput proximale mi. tricipitis brachii

N. radialis

Vasa collateralia radialia

Vasa collateralia media
et R. mi. anconaei

Rr. musculares capitis proximalis
mi. tricipitis brachii

Caput distale mi. tricipitis
et R. muscularis

N. radialis et A. collateralis radialis

Septum intermusculare radiale

M. brachioradialis

N. cutaneus antebrachii dorsalis
et Vasa collateralia radialia

Caput proximale mi. tricipitis brachii

Caput distale mi. tricipitis brachii

Epicondylus ulnaris humeri

Epicondylus radialis humeri

Fig. 3.1 Posterior brachial region and radial nerve channel. Tendon of lateral triceps muscle head obscured by muscles. (From von Lanz and Wachsmuth 1959)

Wilhelm (1986), Mitsunaga and Nakano (1988), Nakamichi and Tschibana (1991) and Wilhelm (1993).

A partial or even a complete paralysis of the forearm muscles innervated by the radial nerve and disturbances of sensibility at the inferior lateral cutaneous brachii nerve, the posterior cutaneous antebrachii nerve and the superficial branch of the radial nerve can be the result (Fig. 3.2a). Irritations of the radial nerve at this site often result in pain radiation into the lateral epicondyle region (TE), into the extension side of the hand (posterior interosseous nerve neuralgia; Wachsmuth and Wilhelm 1967) and into the region of the radial styloid process (so-called radial styloiditis), summarised as radial irritation syndrome (RIS) (cf. Fig. 3.1; Wilhelm 1972, see references of Chap. 1).

Table 3.3 PRKS: localisation of pressure damage	A. Triceps muscle lateral head	13×
	B. Radial nerve hiatus	10×
	C. Combination of A and B	5×
	D. Localisation distal to the hiatus	2×

The fibrous border of the radial nerve hiatus arcade is the next physiological bottleneck, sometimes narrowed even more by transverse fibrous strands of the septum (Fig. 3.3b). In this case there is also a pressure damage of the nerve and pain radiation into these regions without the supraepicondyle and posterior pain area, innervated by the lateral collateral branch of the radial nerve and the anconeus muscle branch. Disturbance of sensibility in this case is only found at the superficial branch of the radial nerve (Fig. 3.3a).

A further quite rare physiological narrowness is found at a fibrous band structure distal to the radial nerve hiatus, stretching between the bases of the brachial muscle and the lateral intermuscular septum of the humeral shaft in low height (Fig. 3.4a).

Myokinetic and sensitive disturbance corresponds to those in radial nerve hiatus compression.

Localisation of pressure damage is demonstrated in Table 3.3.

3.3 Epidemiology

Apart from the author's statistics, there are no other significant publications on the subject; consequently at this point, no definite answer can be given concerning the frequency of PRKS. The occurrence of PRKS can be estimated indirectly, for example, by comparison to the supinator syndrome. This relation was 27:29 in favour of the supinator syndrome between the years 1968 and 1988. This result, however, does not allow for reliable conclusions concerning the prevalence.

Based on patient population, an average age of 45 years (18–70 years) and a preference of the male sex in a ratio of 17:13, as well as a side localisation of 12:18 in favour of the left arm, are seen.

Triggering factors are mainly occupational, acute and chronic overexertion of the triceps muscle in a ratio of 10:20 with special significance of favourable anatomic conditions and variations (Table 3.1).

3.4 Aetiology and Pathogenesis

The most essential triggering causes of PRKS have already been mentioned in the preceding sections and have been presented in Tables 3.1 and 3.2.

- *Four mechanisms of compression were found as the cause of PRKS.*

The *1st compression mechanism* is a relatively narrow triceps muscle portion of origin with the lateral head in longitudinal direction compressing the nerve in the flat spiral sulcus in the case of acute or chronic overexertion.

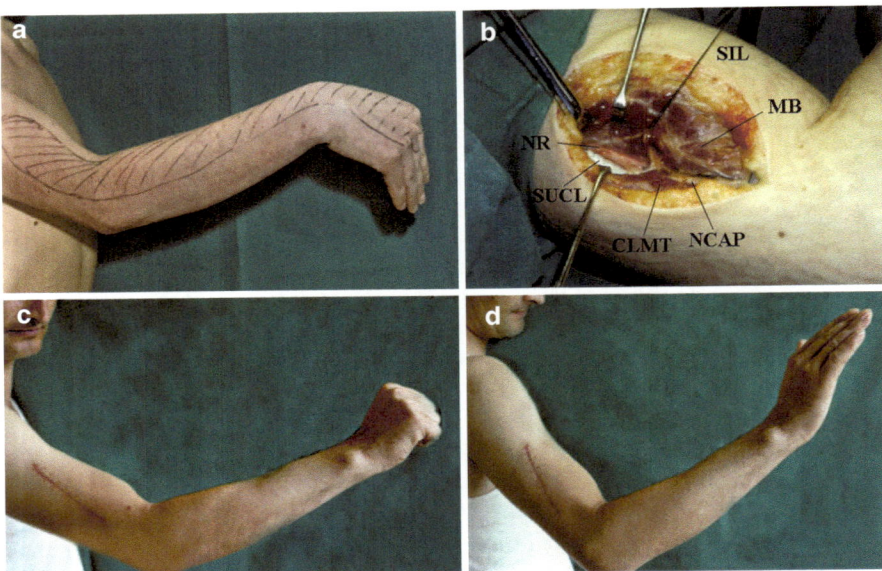

Fig. 3.2 PRKS: *The 1st compression mechanism is caused by the tendinous portion of origin of triceps muscle lateral head proximal to the radial nerve hiatus* (pat. 5). (**a**) Clinical aspect: complete radial paresis with sensibility disorder at the inferior lateral cutaneous brachii nerve, the posterior cutaneous nerve of the forearm and the superficial branch of the radial nerve. (**b**) Presentation of radial nerve and compressing the tendinous portion of triceps muscle lateral head, which still has to be resected (1st compression mechanism) and the hiatus already partly resected. Front border of lateral intermuscular septum (SIL) with black suture; *MB* brachial muscle, *NCAP* posterior cutaneous nerve of the forearm, *CLMT* triceps muscle lateral head, *SUCL* tendinous portion of origin of lateral head, *NR* radial nerve with disturbance of subepineural blood flow and start of indentation (**c**) functional result 8 weeks after surgery: wrist extension (**d**) functional result 5 months after surgery: extension of joint and fingers. (From Wilhelm 1970a, b, c, d)

In our patient population the immediate development of this complete radial paresis was first seen after the sudden stop of a compression air drill, leading to a pressure damage of the nerve due to the sudden contraction of the triceps muscle (Table 3.1, no. 5; Fig. 3.2a; access: Fig. 3.7). If there also is a significant swelling of the nerve, a secondary entrapment of the nerve at the lateral intermuscular septum is also possible.

The 2nd compression mechanism concerns the radial nerve hiatus, functionally being a relatively short osteofibrous channel (Table 3.1, no 29; Fig. 3.3; access Fig. 3.7). Also masses like callus development in the healing of upper arm fracture, haematoma and tumour can lead to a compression of the radial nerve, as under these conditions the nerve is pushed from the inner side to the outer side being pressed against the sharp edge of the hiatus. Inflammatory and noninflammatory swelling of the nerve can also lead to pressure damage.

The 3rd mechanism of compression is a fibrous arcade stretching some centimetres distal to the radial nerve hiatus in the depth from the brachial muscle to the

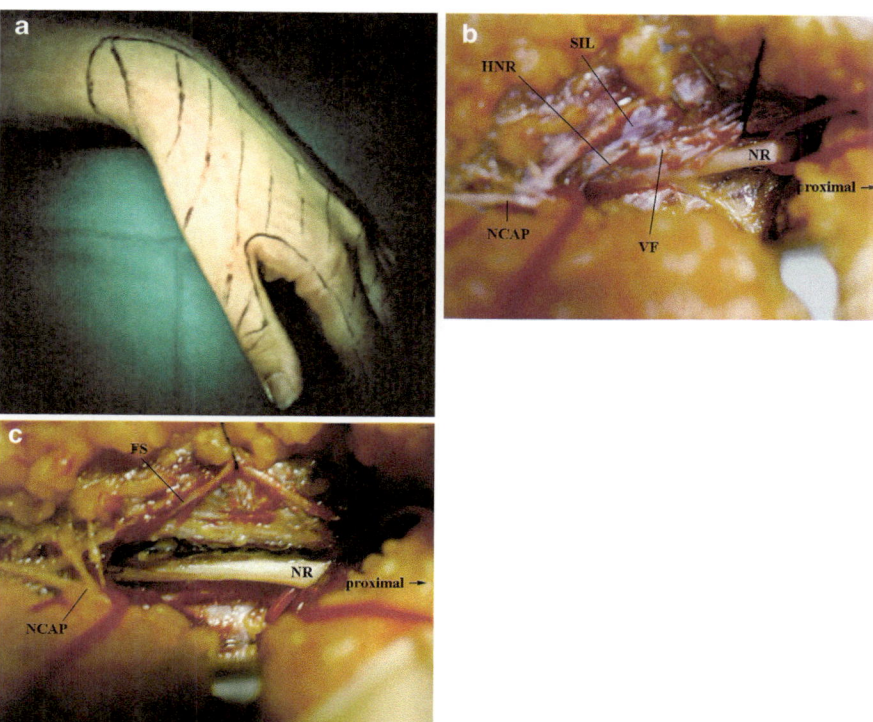

Fig. 3.3 Proximal radial compression syndrome (PRKS): *2nd compression mechanism* (radial nerve compression at the radial nerve hiatus). (**a**) Complete radial paresis with sensibility disorder at the superficial branch of the radial nerve. (**b**) Surgical aspect: preparation of posterior cutaneous nerve of the forearm (*NCAP*) and radial nerve (*NR*), radial nerve hiatus (*HNR*) with fibrous plate in front of HNR with black suture (*VF*; pat. 29), *SIL* lateral intermuscular septum. (**c**) Intraoperative aspect: status post resection of fibrous plate and radial nerve hiatus (pat. 29); intense disturbance of subepineural blood flow and indentation in intermediate section, *NCAP* posterior cutaneous nerve of the forearm, *FS* superficial fascia, marked by black suture upwards; postoperative complete reconstitution of function

septum base, also forming a fibrous channel with the humeral shaft below (Table 3.1, pat. 26; Fig. 3.4a; access: Fig. 3.8a). A ball-shaped callus after upper arm fracture in this patient leads to a complete secondary radial paresis in 5 weeks. After decompression there was a complete functional restitution after 4 1/2 months (Table 3.6).

The radial nerve in the further course of the upper arm can also be damaged between the brachioradial and the brachial muscle by overexertion, for example, by lifting a heavy oven (*4th mechanism of compression*; Fig. 3.5a; *access* Fig. 3.8a).

In this case there was a heavy partial radial paresis. Anamnestically and in checking the course of motion, there was a massive tension of the above-mentioned muscles as cause of this damage; the radial nerve was suddenly pressed in anterior direction with pressure damage by crossing structures, mostly fibrous fibres and vessels at

Fig. 3.4 Proximal radial compression syndrome (PRKS): *3rd compression mechanism*: fibrous arcade stretching distally of radial nerve hiatus in the depth of the brachial muscle to septum base forming an osteofibrous channel together with the humeral shaft. (**a**) Intraoperative aspect: complete secondary paresis with disturbance of sensibility at the radial nerve superficial branch caused by a tight fibrous plate (*FP*) between brachial muscle (*MB*) and lateral intermuscular septum (*SIL*); *NCAP* posterior cutaneous nerve of the forearm; *NR* radial nerve. (**b**) Intraoperative aspect: after resection of fibrous plate a disturbance of subepineural blood flow and an indentation is seen (pat. 26)

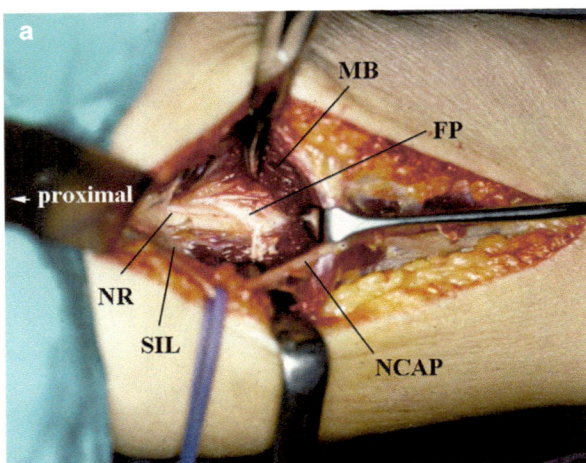

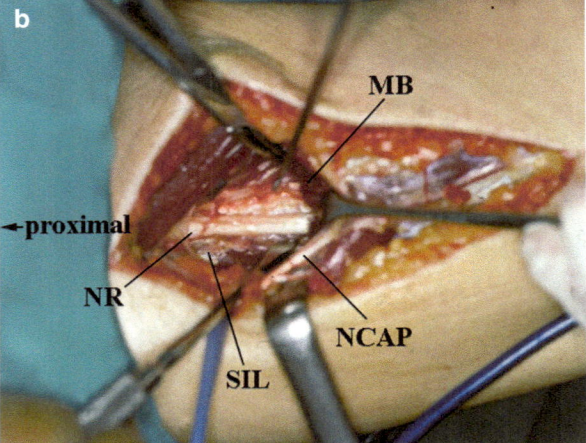

several sites of a fascicle in the sense of an axonotmesis, that is, preserving the continuity of the nerve sheath. These injuries at the side of a fascicle are called *sandglass-shaped constriction*. Several following lesions should be called *segmentations*.

The first term is a little misleading, as in contrast to the regular function of a sandglass, the constriction in this injury is caused by distortion of the nerve stumps or segments and in many cases is not permeable for the sprouting neurites any more, as already proved in the clinical course after waiting longer, by histological examinations. The proximal stump of the nerve develops a neuroma, whereas degenerative changes predominate in the distal area.

In a fresh injury this result can only be corrected by immediate indication for revision of the nerve with derotation of the nerve stumps or even the single segments, then they have to be connected to neighbouring structures by most delicate atraumatic sutures in order to prevent a new torsion of the segments (Fig. 3.5a). Depending on the extent of the findings, additionally an immobilisation for several weeks is necessary.

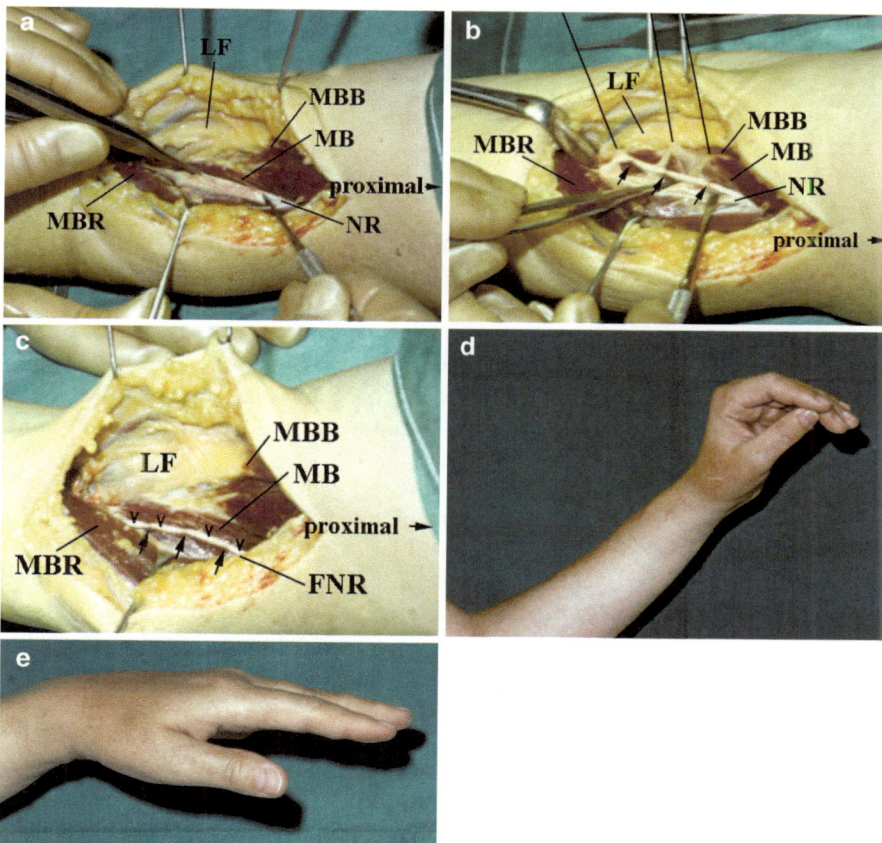

Fig. 3.5 Proximal radial compression syndrome (PRKS): *4th compression mechanism* (pressure damage of radial nerve between brachioradial muscle and brachial muscle due to overexertion in this case causing segmentation or torsion of a motoric neurofascicle). (**a**) Intraoperative aspect: preparation of radial nerve in proximal section of anterior radial channel due to complete paralysis of finger and thumb extensors as well as ECU; partial paresis of radiodorsal muscles of the hand. Locally subepineural haematoma of 3 cm at epicondyle line. *NR* radial nerve, *MBR* brachioradial muscle, *LF* bicipital aponeurosis, *MBB* biceps muscle, *MB* brachial muscle (pat. not shown on table). (**b**) Intraoperative aspect: after epineurolysis at the strongest fascicle three cases of crushing with distance of 1–1.5 cm are found, segments being connected only by perineural tube. Also segments are contorted at the sites of the hourglass-shaped constrictions (*arrows*). Crossing structures marked by *black lines*. *NR* radial nerve, *MBR* brachioradial muscle, *LF* bicipital aponeurosis, *MBB* biceps muscle, *MB* brachial muscle; (**c**) intraoperative aspect: crossing structures are resected for therapeutic reasons, segments are derotated and fixated to brachial muscle with delicate sutures to prevent recurrence of torsion. *FNR* fascicle of radial nerve, *MBR* brachioradial muscle, *LF* bicipital aponeurosis, *MBB* biceps muscle, *MB* brachial muscle, (**d** and **e**) functional result after 5 months. (From Wilhelm 1976)

Wilhelm (1976), Burn and Lister (1984), Yamamoto et al. (2000), Yongwei et al. (2003) and Wasmeier et al. (2004) described these mono- and polyfascicular radial lesions at the upper arm.

A simple pressure damage of the radial nerve between the brachioradial muscle and brachial muscle in the shape of an indentation has been reported by Lee et al. (2006).

3.5   Diagnostics

Anamnesis is most important in diagnostics of a proximal radial compression syndrome in order to rule out exogenous factors and to receive hints at the presentation of an acute or chronic endogenous nerve damage. Here mainly diagnosis of an occupational or sports stress, mainly on the function of the triceps muscle, is essential, apart from the duration of trauma and the time of radial paresis.

A detailed analysis of the motion pattern in question is next, as well as an examination of the muscles innervated by the radial nerve and the sensibility disorders found as well as the pain localisation (Table 3.4).

If the forearm muscles innervated by the radial nerve are paralysed, there is a carpoptosis and a disappearance of the brachioradial bulging in flexion of the elbow joint as well as sensibility disorders at the inferior lateral cutaneous brachial nerve, the posterior antebrachii cutaneous nerve and the superficial branch of the radial nerve (Fig. 3.2). In many cases this is also true for pain areas in the lateral epicondyle region (tennis elbow), in the back of the hand (neuralgia of the posterior interosseous nerve) and above the radial styloid process (radial styloiditis), especially in minor pressure damage (Table 3.4).

In case there is only disturbance of sensibility of the superficial radial nerve branch and apart from a pain area in the anterior section of the lateral epicondyle region there also is neuralgia of the posterior interosseous nerve, pressure damage is found at either the radial nerve hiatus or the distally adjacent short osteofibrous channel, formed by the humeral shaft and a fibrous plate, or a compression of the nerve in the medial section of the radial tunnel and the supinator gap (tennis elbow)

Table 3.4 Preoperative findings:$N_{path.} = 30$		
A. Motor function		
Complete pareses		14×
Partial pareses		8×
Reduction of crude strength (PRIS)[a]		8×
B. Sensibility disorders		
N. radialis: Hoffmann-Tinel		27×
N. cutaneus brachii posterior		5×
N. cutaneus antebrachii posterior		20×
R. superficialis ni. radialis		20×
C. Pain regions		
Lateral epicondyle		15×
Proc. styl. radii		4×
Back of hand (interosseous neuralgia)		6×

[a]Proximal radial irritation syndrome

(Figs. 3.3a and 3.4a). In this case a possible "double crush nerve lesion" has to be checked diligently.

Should anamnesis hint at a fracture of the humeral shaft or at infectious or tumourous processes, corresponding x-rays should be done, of course.

Finally, a neurological exam follows; it should be performed directly after the development of acute paresis to prevent the necessity of a secondary suture or bridging by nerve transplant in mono- or polyfascicular segmentation.

Apart from exogenous pressure damage, primary radial injury by upper arm fracture and tumour-caused compression in the gap between the brachial and the brachioradial muscles have to be considered in *differential diagnosis.*

An isolated tennis elbow, not developed in the context of RIS as "double crush nerve lesion", has to be noted as well as the symptom complex of a thoracic inlet syndrome (TIS), as one can see in Table 3.1 chronic edema in 4 out of 30 cases also favoured the nerve compression as a causal effect.

Pathogenetic significance of such chronic edema was already clinically and histologically found to be the cause of idiopathic distal median compression in 1985 (Wilhelm and Wilhelm 1985; Fig. 5.1).

In order to be complete, the "myokinetic" supinator syndrome has to be mentioned, where only function of the brachioradial muscle and both radial extensors remains. In this case the joint can only be extended with simultaneous deviation of the hand in radial direction, as the ulnar carpi extensor muscle is paralysed as well. At the same time there is complete loss of finger extension in all MP joints, whereas extension in the interphalangeal joints is preserved, as this function is taken over by the lumbrical muscles innervated by the ulnar nerve.

In this supinator syndrome there frequently is pressure pain at the entry and exit of the supinator channel, also above the intramuscular course of the radial nerve, which can additionally be compressed at diverse sites (Figs. 1.8 and 1.9). Pain can radiate in direction of the lateral epicondyle and proximally to the upper arm, distally to the back of the hand and the MP joints of the fingers (neuralgia of posterior interosseous nerve) (Fig. 1.3).

Finally it has to be mentioned that sensibility disorder at the superficial radial branch can also result from a compression of this nerve between the tendons of the brachioradial muscle and the long radial carpi extensor muscle (Wartenberg syndrome, 1954). Diagnosis is simple as there is local pressure pain and deterioration of pain by pronation of the forearm, closing the narrowness and the adjacent rims of the muscles compressing the superficial radial branch. In supination, however, the tendon rims move divergently, the narrowness opens and an improvement of pain develops.

3.6 Classification

Reviewing our patient population, we found that regeneration time in complete paresis by no means depends on the duration of prior patient history but entirely on the severity of the local compression damage or the nerve lesion. Thus, complete paresis was subdivided into those with most severe local changes (+++: pat. 4;

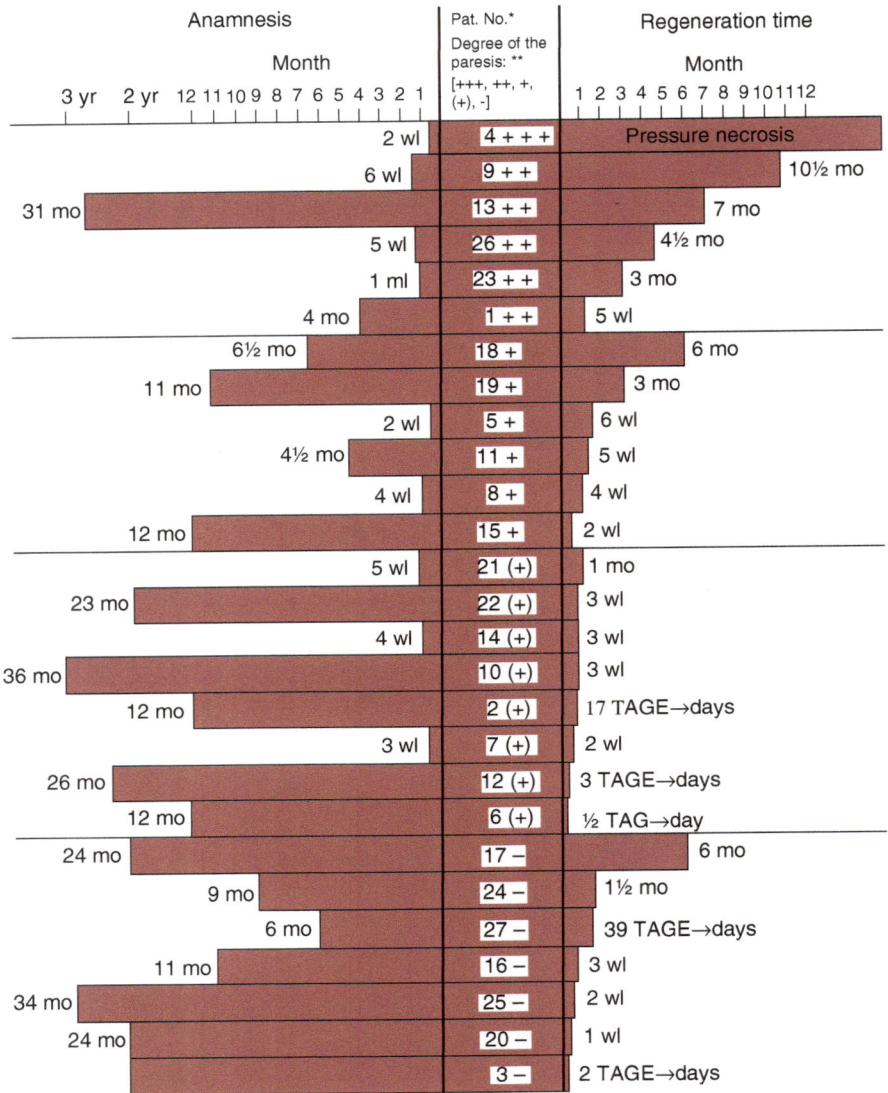

*The patients 28, 29 [+] and 30 [-] with a anamnesis of 8,3 resp. 22 month are not taken into consideration, as the time of regeneration could not be elicited anymore.
**Classification see section 3.6
***Further seven pats. could not be judged, as all documents were destroyed. The total number of surgically treated pats. consequently amounted to 37.

Fig. 3.6 PRKS: N_p (1969–1990), $N_{op} = 30$ results

radial nerve necrosis), with severe (++: pats. 9, 13, 26, 23, 1), minor (+: pats. 18, 19, 5, 11, 8, 15, 28, 29) and slight (+: pats. 21, 22, 14, 10, 2, 7, 12, 6) degree of change. Ongoing proximal radial irritation syndromes were also marked (−) (Fig. 3.6).

3.7 Therapy

3.7.1 Conservative Treatment

Conservative treatment will only succeed in a single overuse of the triceps muscle with consecutive impairment of crude strength and sensibility disorder, as well as in sudden appearance of a radial irritation syndrome. In both cases there is focus on therapeutic relief of the triceps muscle by protection and immediate discontinuation or removal of the triggering causes with consecutive information. The patient also needs to know any flexion in the elbow joint, especially when using force will lengthen the recovery time. A dorsal upper arm plastic cast in flexion of the elbow joint of 0-30-0° is mainly advisable in stronger pain and also for the night.

Conservative treatment can also be considered in single overexertion of the triceps muscle with consecutive complete or partial paresis until examinations are completed. In chronic trauma conservative treatment should also be attempted until examinations are completed and urgent pretreatment has been finished.

3.7.1.1 Indications for Conservative Treatment

1. *Acute trauma* with single overexertion of the triceps muscle, reduction of crude strength and sensibility disorder (neurological exam!)
   (a) Relief of triceps muscle by protection, discontinuation of triggering cause
   (b) Anti-inflammatory medication if needed
2. *Single overexertion of triceps muscle* with complete and partial paresis
   (a) Conservative therapy until completion of neurological exam, necessary earlier than after 3 days
   (b) Surgical revision of proximal radial channel in 1 week in order to treat mono- or multifascicular nerve constriction best, by derotation and fixation of segments
3. *Chronic Trauma*
   (a) Conservative therapy until completion of examinations and possibly necessary urgent pretreatment
   (b) Check of workplace and motion pattern of the arm affected
   (c) Pretreatment of additional factors (focal toxicity, metabolic disorder)—alcohol abuse!
   (d) Surgical revision of radial nerve after neurological exam

3.7.2 Surgical Treatment

Indications for surgical therapy are shown in Table 3.5.

Technique of PRKS decompression and surgical treatment of radial injury at the bicipital sulcus between brachial muscle and brachioradial muscle, possible in differential diagnosis (cf. below).

Informed Patient Consent
• Explanation of possible compression mechanisms and surgical principles also mentioning the possibility of combined procedures, such as resection of an older

Table 3.5 PRKS: indications of surgery

A. Acute pareses, after conservative treatment	4×
B. Pareses due to chronic trauma	15×
C. Pareses in inflammatory process	3×
D. Secondary pareses in course of healing fracture	8×
Surgical procedures	30×

constriction followed by primary nerve coadaptation or interfascicular nerve transplant and immobilisation for 3 weeks. This also applies to compression of the radial nerve in the anterior area of the radial channel.

- In radial paresis by tumour injury of the outer nerve sheath in preparation should be mentioned as well.
- Time of surgery 60–90 min, depending on local findings.
- Success rate for treatment of proximal radial compression syndrome is excellent, apart from severe pressure damage in the sense of nerve necrosis. Replacement of function by radial graft is possible.
- Remaining complaints, especially in independently persisting areas of disturbance at the neck, shoulder and arm.
- Usual postoperative complications like swelling of soft tissue, bleeding and infections

Instruments
- Instruments for hand surgery
- Bipolar electric coagulation
- Magnifying glasses or microscope for surgery

Anaesthesia and Positioning
- Upper or lower plexus anaesthesia or intubation
- Position on the back
- Bandaging of arm towards the trunk and application of controlled upper arm partial deprivation of blood supply. Cuff pressure between 200 and max. 300 mmHg
- Positioning of arm slightly flexed on a cloth padding

3.7.2.1 Decompression of Radial Nerve at the Tendinous Origin of the Lateral Head of the Triceps Muscle and the Radial Nerve Hiatus (Compression Mechanisms 1, 2 and 3)

An extreme deprivation of blood supply is needed for preparation of the radial nerve. After longitudinal incision at the outer side of the upper arm in extension of the supraepicondylar crista (access: Fig. 3.7), the fascia behind the lateral intermuscular septum and the exit of the posterior antebrachii cutaneous nerve are prepared. The latter is the *leading structure* for identification of the radial nerve between the front rim of the triceps muscle lateral head and the lateral intermuscular septum.

This cutaneous nerve in the subcutis is looked for and then followed in proximal direction until it exits from the superficial fascia. From here the upper arm fascia is first incised longitudinally between the front rim of the triceps muscle and the lateral intermuscular septum diligently preserving the cutaneous nerve and its accompanying vessels. After pulling aside the triceps bulge, you see the cutaneous nerve

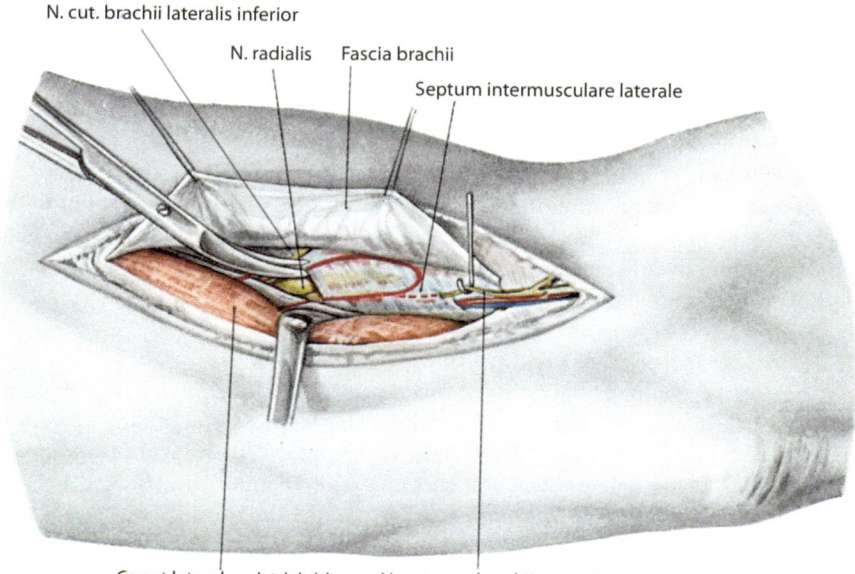

N. cut. brachii lateralis inferior

N. radialis   Fascia brachii

Septum intermusculare laterale

Caput laterale mi. tricipitis   N. cut. antebrachii posterior

Fig. 3.7 Decompression of radial nerve in proximal radial compression syndrome according to Wilhelm. Preparation of posterior cutaneous nerve of the forearm (leading structure) in proximal direction and dissection of the radial nerve (*hatched line*). *Red lines*: resection of the tendinous portion of origin of triceps muscle lateral head along the course of the radial nerve and the radial nerve hiatus. (From Wilhelm, see Mittelbach 1972)

at the back rim of the septum, which can also be covered by a superficial layer of the septum as presented in Fig. 3.7. This structure is incised in longitudinal direction up to the level of the radial nerve hiatus. After pulling aside the triceps bulge, you see the radial nerve entering the hiatus and proximally the posterior antebrachii cutaneous nerve and in the depth the tendinous portion of origin of the triceps muscle lateral head. It is resected above the transverse course of the radial nerve, as it is *responsible for the first compression mechanism*. Afterwards the radial nerve is examined diligently in this area, especially taking care of existence or lack of subepineural blood supply and other consequences of compression.

3.7.2.2 Resection of Radial Nerve Hiatus
Then the *hiatus, responsible for the second mechanism of compression*, is opened above the radial nerve in anterior direction and resected extensively. Always keep in mind whether the nerve additionally is damaged by a fibrous compressive structure (Fig. 3.3b).

3.7.2.3 Resection of Fibrous Arcade
Under regular conditions, the nerve should also be revised distal to the septum, as it can rarely be damaged by crossing fibrous strands in this area (*3rd compression mechanism*; Fig. 3.4).

Rebasing of a radial nerve with pressure damage is only necessary in infectious process or in major scarring, as well as in changes of the radial nerve sulcus caused by fractures.

A redon drainage is placed after control of haemorrhage and wound closure layer by layer follows. The superficial fascia is closed by loosely adapting sutures. In decompression of RIS a simple compressive dressing suffices for postoperative treatment. An upper arm plastic cast supported by a dynamic radial splint in order to relieve the paralysed forearm muscles is necessary in partial and complete paresis for preventing overdistension of the paralysed forearm muscles.

Depending on the secretion, redon drainage is removed after 1–2 days.

3.7.2.4 Intraoperative Findings

More severe pressure damages of the radial nerve were found in 6 out of 30 patients (Table 3.6). It was also possible to localise the compression damage macroscopically in the remaining cases (Table 3.6). In 13 out of 30 surgical procedures, the localisation of the damage was the crossing of the lateral triceps head tendinous portion of origin (*1st compression mechanism*), and in ten cases it was the area of the radial nerve hiatus (*2nd compression mechanism*). Five patients showed a combination of both pressure localisations, while compression damage of the radial nerve distal to the hiatus was only registered twice (*3rd compression mechanism*). Further on the radial nerve can be damaged by pressure at the lateral bicipital sulcus caused by sudden muscle contractions, where the nerve is suddenly relocated in anterior direction and pressed against crossing structures (vessels and fibres). Mono- and polyfascicular compression lesion results (*4th compression mechanism*; Fig. 3.5, no table).

Most macroscopic changes were found intraoperatively in the shape of indentations at the lateral head of the triceps muscle and the radial nerve hiatus in about half of the operations (Table 3.6). Constriction ring-shaped compressions were only seen at the hiatus. Anatomic variations at the hiatus were also responsible for compression of the radial nerve at this place, but they can also work as the sole source of compression. The most severe compression in the shape of an extended necrosis at the lateral tricipital head and the hiatus was only found once (Fig. 3.6). The radial replacement plastic planned taking into account local findings and age of the patient was not agreed to, unfortunately.

Table 3.6 PRKS: intraoperative findings: $N_{op} = 30$

A. Dimpling (Caput laterale and hiatus of radial nerve) and disturbance of subepineural blood flow (N_p: 2, 3, 5, 7, 8, 10, 11, 14, 16, 18, 19, 20, 26, 28, 29)[a]	15×
B. Constriction ring (hiatus of radial nerve) (N_p: 1, 7, 9, 12, 13, 17)[a]	6×
C. Thickening of epineurium (N_p: 1, 5, 7)[a]	3×
D. Scarry embedding (N_p: 1, 12, 22, 23, 29)[a]	5×
E. Pressure necrosis (Caput laterale and hiatus of radial nerve) (N_p: 4)[a]	1×
F. Radial nerve o. k. Macroscopically: disturbance of the intraneural flow (N_p: 6, 15)[a]	2×
G. Anatomic variety (N_p: 8, 10, 18, 20, 29, 30)	6×

[a]Numbers refer of corresponding numbers of Table 3.1

Epineural thickening was seen in three patients, whereas scarry embedding of the radial nerve was seen in 26 patients. Only 4 out of 30 patients did show no macroscopic pathological findings after decompression of the radial nerve; here a disturbance of the intraneural flow was supposed to be the cause of the complaints. Anatomic variations were found in seven cases.

3.7.2.5 Surgical Treatment by Decompression of Radial Nerve in Lateral Bicipital Fissure

The radial nerve can be compressed not only by sudden contraction of the brachioradial, brachial and biceps brachii muscles at the lateral bicipital sulcus but also by tumour development. Even though the latter only has to be accounted for in differential diagnosis of PRKS, they are described here as their symptoms can resemble those of the 3rd and 4th compression mechanism (Fig. 3.9a; access: Fig. 3.8a).

A longitudinal incision at the lateral bicipital sulcus, which can possibly be extended to the angle of the elbow in a bow shape, noticing the distal flexion crease of the joint (Fig. 3.8a; dotted line; serves as access). Then the superficial fascia is opened along the medial rim of the cephalic vein and also extended in a bow shape at the angle of the elbow. Also the exit of the lateral cutaneous antebrachii nerve has to be preserved (Fig. 3.8b). Then the radial nerve is prepared and inspected in the depth between the brachioradial and brachial muscles, especially taking notice of crossing structures (Figs. 3.8c).

In single or multiple constrictions (segmentations) further proceeding primarily depends on the age of injury. In fresh injury derotation of the segments is recommended; they have to be fixed to neighbouring structures (brachial muscle) by fine atraumatic sutures in order to prevent repetitive rotation. In older injury depending on the damage, either resection of the scarred constriction ring with suture following or extensive resection with defect bridging by nerve transplant has to be performed. In all cases finally immobilisation of the arm in a plastic upper arm splint in slight flexion of the elbow joint in 0-30-0° is necessary in combination with an additional supplementation by a dynamic radial cast.

In the tumour lesion the nerve is cautiously dissected and the tumour is removed. In this case a longitudinal incision of the epineurium is only necessary in severe pressure damage with massive reduction of nerve diameter.

3.8   Results

Postoperative results are summarised in Fig. 3.6 and in Table 3.7. Here it is seen that complete and incomplete paresis as well as irritation syndromes (−) vanished in 29 out of 30 cases. Only one patient (pat. 9, no. 4) with an extensive pressure necrosis did not get back function as he did not agree to the radial graft needed.

In patients 28 and 29 paresis subsided completely. Comments on duration of regeneration can however not be made any more. This is also true for a patient (30) with RIS.

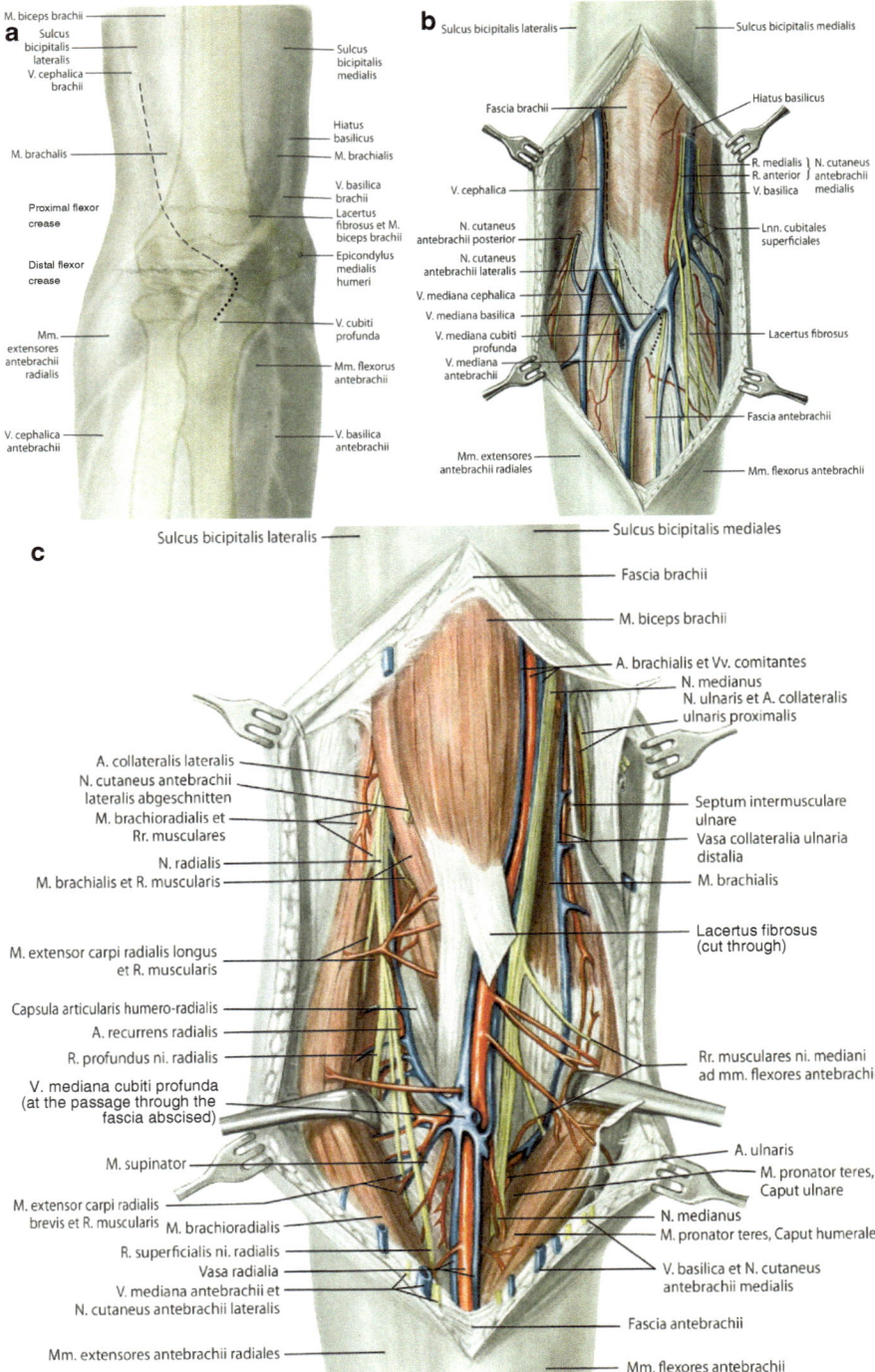

Fig. 3.8 Surgical approach in compression of radial nerve in the distal half of the upper arm: (**a**) planning of skin incision, (**b**) planning of fascia incision, (**c**) schematic surgical site of radial nerve at the upper arm. (Taken from von Lanz and Wachsmuth 1959)

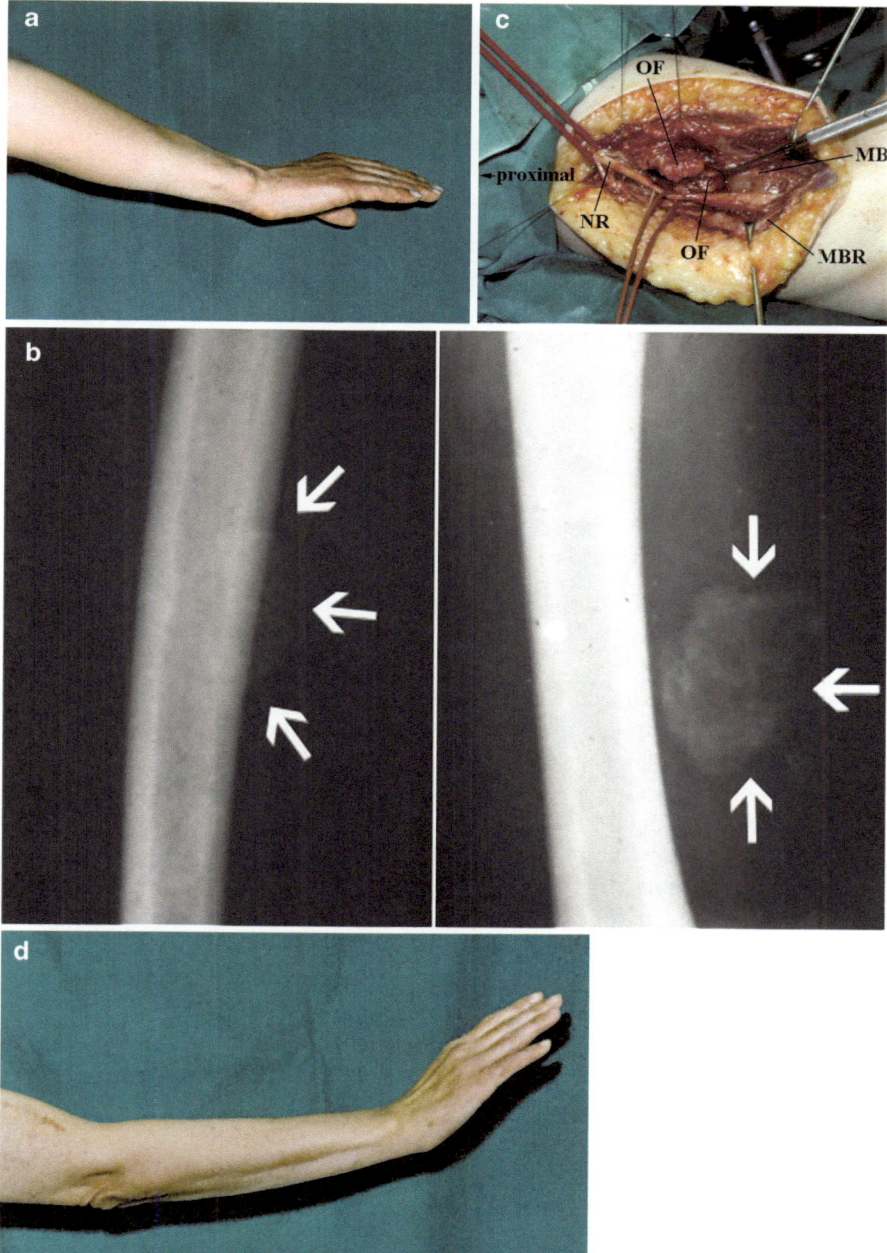

Fig. 3.9 Partial radial paresis of the right upper extremity caused by the tumour at the lateral bicipital sulcus, (**a**) preoperative finding, (**b**) radiologically big osseous formation (histological osteofibroma, limitation by *white arrows*), (**c**) intraoperative site: compression of radial nerve (*NR*) by the tumour grown in semi-circle (*OF*); nerve already loosened from the sulcus of the tumour (spatula); *MB* brachial muscle; *MBR* brachioradial muscle, (**d**) postoperative result after 4 months

Table 3.7 Postoperative results: $N_p = 27/(30)$

A. *Motor function*	
Complete restitution of pareses	13×
Complete paresis due to pressure damage[a]	1×
Complete restoration of partial pareses	8×
Recovery of crude strength	17×
Improvement of crude strength	2×
Lack of crude strength[a]	1×
B. *Sensibility Disorders*	
N. radialis: Hoffmann-Tinel	1×
Hoffmann-Tinel, slight	2×
N. cutaneus brachii posterior	1×
N. cutaneus antebrachii posterior	1×
R. superficialis ni. radialis	2× (+1×)[b]
C. *Pain regions*	
Lateral epicondyle region	1× (+2×)[b]
Styloid process of radius	0 (+1×)[b]
Back of hand (interosseous neuralgia)	0 (+1×)[b]

Individual postoperative results in patients 28, 29 and 30 are not taken into account, as documentation is missing
[a] Cf. Fig. 3.6, no. 1
[b] Findings in brackets are due to an independently existing tennis elbow

As mentioned above, the duration of regeneration only depended on the severity of local findings. Thus, complete paresis with severe compression damage showed the longest time of regeneration, whereas identical paresis with less lesion recuperated in much less time. In partial paresis the duration of regeneration was 12 h to 1 month maximum!

In irritation syndrome symptoms receded in 2 days to 1½ months max., in one case only after 6 months (Fig. 3.6).

Control of the velocity of nerve conduction is necessary for judging postoperative results. The example shown in Fig. 3.10 preoperatively shows a velocity of nerve conduction of only 33.3 m/s and 5 weeks after surgery shows a quite normal level of 46.0 m/s (Fig. 3.6, pat. 27).

3.9   Mistakes, Dangers and Complications

In diligent anamnesis and examination of the entire upper extremity, in timely neurological exam and recognition of therapeutic indications (Table 3.7), there should be no mistakes with consequences—only if the radial nerve was directly dissected without primary preparation of its indicating structure (posterior cutaneous nerve of the forearm). In this case, apart from the danger of severe traumatisation of tissue, there is the risk of injuring nervous structures, such as the cutaneous nerve mentioned, but also of the radial nerve itself. Mistakes can also arise from not resecting the lateral triceps muscle tendinous portion of origin even though a macroscopically

Fig. 3.10 Pre- and postoperative control (*below*) and velocity of neural flow

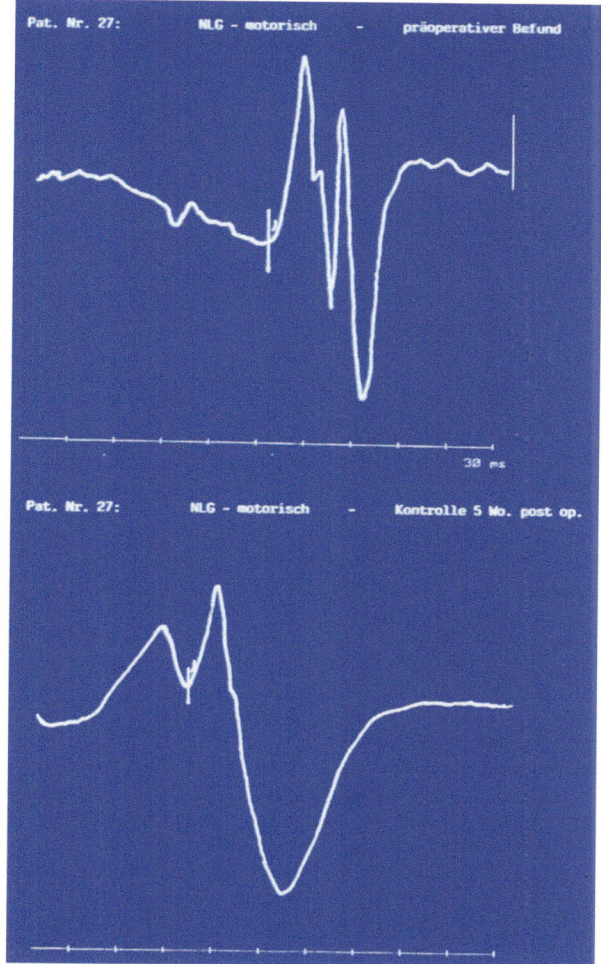

discernible pressure damage at the radial nerve hiatus exists, even though an exact anamnesis would have called for a massive overexertion of the triceps muscle. In case of doubt, a radial nerve decompression should be performed at the first and second pressure location. If there are no striking signs of compression here, the course of the nerve also has to be revised distal to the hiatus.

In acute constriction injury revision of the nerve basically has to be undertaken immediately, that is, during the first week in order to enable the patient to receive the most simple treatment, being derotation with additional fixation of segments. In all cases where revision was postponed, patients had to be prepared for resection of the compression followed by suture or even a nerve transplant. The latter therapeutic methods are also applied in older constrictions. Yongwei et al. (2003) were able to treat only 3 out of 8 patients by epineurolysis as they showed only slight constriction, one case failed. The remaining five patients needed resection of the constriction followed by nerve suture in two cases and nerve transplantation in three cases.

Postoperative swelling of soft tissue can be prevented by the removal of drainage only after recession of secretion and first change of dressing only after disappearance of edema. Postoperative infections can mostly be prevented if the surgical site is disinfected and prepared according to the principles of hand surgery (washing and application of 30 % alcohol dressing).

References

Burn J, Lister G (1984) Localized constrictive radial neuropathy in the absence of extrinsic compression: three cases. J Hand surg 9:99–103

Gowers WR (1892) quoted acc. to Sunderland S (1978) Nerves and nerve injuries, 2nd edn. Churchill Livingstone, Edinburgh, p S822

Lanz T von, Wachsmuth W (1959) Praktische Anatomie [Practical anatomy], Band 1, Teil 3: Arm. Springer, Berlin, pp S127–S129

Lee YK, Kim YI, Choy WS (2006) Radial nerve compression between the brachialis and brachioradialis muscles in a manual worker: a case report. J Hand Surg 31 A:744–746

Lotem M, Fried A, Levy M, Solzi P, Najenson T, Nathian H (1971) Radial palsy following muscular effort. J Bone Joint Surg 53 B:500–506

Lubahn JD, Lister G (1983) Familial radial nerve entrapment syndrome. J Hand Surg 8:297–299

Manske PR (1977) Compression of the radial nerve by the triceps muscle: case report. J Bone Joint Surg 59 A:835–836

Mitsunaga MM, Nakano K (1988) High radial nerve palsy following strenuous muscular activity. Clin Orthop 234:39–42

Mittelbach HR (1972) Nervendruckschäden [Nerve damage by pressure]. In: Wachsmuth W, Wilhelm A (Hrsg) Die Operationen an der Hand. In: Zenker R, Heberer G, Hegemann G (Hrsg) Allgemeine und spezielle chirurgische Operationslehre, Bd X/3. Springer, Berlin/Heidelberg/New York, pp S254–S263

Nakamichi KI, Tschibana S (1991) Radial nerve entrapment by the lateral head of triceps. J Hand Surg 16 A:748–750

Tackmann W, Richter H P, Stöhr M (1989) Kompressionssyndrome peripherer Nerven [Compression syndromes of peripheral nerves]. Springer, Berlin/Heidelberg, p S272

Wartenberg R (1954) Digitalgia paraesthetica and gonyalgia paraestetica. Neurology (Minneap) 4:102

Wachsmuth W, Wilhelm A (1967) Zur Ätiologie, Diagnose und Behandlung unklarer Schmerzzustände an der Handwurzel [Etiology, diagnosis, and treatment of obscure pain syndromes at the wrist]. Mschr Unfallheilk 10:89–110

Wasmeier C, Pfadenhauer K, Kalbarzcyk H, Becker T, Rösler A (2004) Subakutes proximales Engpasssyndrom des Nervus radialis im Hiatus radialis [Subacute proximal entrapment syndrome of radial nerve at the radial hiatus]. Nervenarzt 75(8):780–784

Wilhelm A (1970a) Neues über Druckschäden des Nervus ulnaris und Nervus radialis [Update on pressure damage of ulnar and radial nerve]. Vortrag, gehalten am 30.05.1970 auf dem 11. Handchirurgischen Symposium in Köln

Wilhelm A (1970b) Das Radialis-Irritationssyndrom (Epicondylitis humeri radialis, Styloiditis radii und Neuralgie des Nervus interosseous dorsalis) [The Radial irritation syndrome (Radial humeral epicondylitis, radial styloiditis, and neuralgia of dorsal interosseous nerve)]. Vortrag, gehalten am 30.05.1970 auf dem 11. Handchirurgischen Symposium in Köln [Lecture given on May 30th 1970 at the 11th congress of hand surgery in Cologne, Germany]

Wilhelm A (1970c) Das Radialisirritationssyndrom [The Radial Irritation Syndrome]. Handchirurgie 2:139–142

Wilhelm A (1970d) Neues über Druckschäden des Nervus ulnaris und Nervus radialis [Update on pressure damages at the ulnar and the radial nerve]. Handchirurgie 2:143–146

Wilhelm A (1972) Die Eingriffe der Schmerzausschaltung durch Denervierung [surgery for Elemination of Pain by Denervation]. In: Wachsmuth W, Wilhelm A (Hrsg.) Die Operationen an der Hand. In: Zenker R, Heberer G, Hegemann G (Hrsg.): Allgemeine und spezielle Operationslehre. Band X, Teil III, Springer Berlin Heidelberg, S264–285

Wilhelm A (1976) Radialiskompressionssyndrome – Über einen weiteren neuen Druckmechanismus des N. radialis [Radial compression syndromes- on a further new pressure mechanism of the radial nerve]. Handchirurgie 8:113–116

Wilhelm A (1986) Nervenkompressionssyndrome der oberen Extremität unter Berücksichtigung der Zugangswege [Nerve compression syndromes of the upper extremity in consideration of the access]. In: Buck-Gramcko D, Nigst H (Hrsg) Bibliothek für Handchirurgie. Hippokrates, Stuttgart, pp S43–S63

Wilhelm A (1993) The proximal radial nerve compression syndrome. In: Tubiana R (ed) The hand, vol IV. Saunders, Philadelphia, pp 390–399

Wilhelm A, Suden R (1985) Das proximale Radialiskompressionssyndrom (PRKS). Behandlung und Ergebnisse [The proximal radial compression syndrome (PRKS). Treatment and results]. Handchirurgie 17:219–224

Wilhelm A, Wilhelm F (1985) Das Thoracic outlet-Syndrom und seine Bedeutung für die Chirurgie der Hand (Zur Ätiologie und Pathogenese der Epicondylitis, Tendovaginitis, Medianuskompression und trophischen Störungen) [the thoracic-outlet-syndrome and its significance in hand surgery (etiology and pathogenesis of epicondylitias, tendovaginitis, median compression, and trophic disturbance)]. Handchir Mikrochir Plast Chir 17:173–187

Yamamoto S, Nagano A, Mikami Y, Tajiri Y (2000) Multiple constrictions of the radial nerve without external compression. J Hand Surg 25 A:134–137

Yongwei P, Guonglei T, Jianing W, Shuhuan W, Qingtai L, Wen T (2003) Nontraumatic paralysis of the radial nerve with multiple constrictions. J Hand Surg 28A:199–205

The Controversial Pain Syndrome of the Shoulder Joint (So-Called Coracoiditis): Pathogenesis and Treatment of Resistant Cases

4

Contents

4.1 Introduction.. 83
4.2 Surgically Relevant Anatomy and Physiology................................. 84
4.3 Epidemiology... 88
4.4 Etiology and Pathogenesis 88
4.5 Diagnostics.. 89
4.6 Classification... 92
4.7 Indications and Contraindications... 92
4.8 Therapy 93
    4.8.1 Technique of Partial Upper Frontal Shoulder Quadrant Denervation of the
        Shoulder Joint According to Wilhelm 93
    4.8.2 Technique of Complete Temporary Pain Elimination at the Shoulder Joint
        According to Wilhelm... 95
4.9 Results.. 98
4.10 Mistakes, Dangers and Complications... 98
References... 98

4.1 Introduction

The region of the shoulder joint is a preferred localisation of diverse causes of pain. These concerns not only solely local but also further proximal and sometimes also distally situated pathological changes in the shape of irritation and compression of the brachial plexus including its origins from C4-Th 1 and peripheral nerves.

In the first case, apart from arthrotic and arthritic as well as rheumatic changes of the shoulder and acromioclavicular joint, mainly diseases of the rotator cuff, summarised under the term *humeroscapular periarthritis,* are found. This includes affections of the subacromial, the subdeltoid and the subcoracoid bursa, as well as the adhesive capsulitis, called *"frozen shoulder"*. Up to now, the so-called coracoiditis was included as well, supposing this pathology is also a tendinopathy. *This is not the case*, however, as this localisation of pain mainly occurs in foraminal stenosis

(C4-C7), thoracic outlet syndrome (TOS) and CRPS I, being treated by conservative or surgical therapy of these syndromes.

In the second case, it is pain radiation caused by proximal compression of the plexus roots mentioned (foramen stenosis) and the brachial plexus at the thoracic outlet (TOS and Sudeck's dystrophy), whereas distal pressure damage occurs at the three main nerve trunks. The carpal tunnel syndrome is an example, known for long. In individual cases, some patients mainly complain about pain of the neck and discomfort radiating into the frontal upper shoulder region. These reactions can also be provoked by palpatory examination of the median nerve at the rascetta. The anterior thoracic nerve together with an articular branch of the stellate ganglion serves for pain projection, as they arise from the same cervical segments (C6-C8) as the median nerve. Similar reactions can also be triggered by a compression of the deep radial branch at the supinator gap, also possibly causing pain radiation into the lateral epicondyle area (TE) and the extension side of the wrist (neuralgia of the posterior interosseous nerve; Wachsmuth and Wilhelm 1967). A corresponding compression of the ulnar nerve at the ulnar nerve sulcus caused pain in extreme flexion and by the so-called flexion test (Wachsmuth and Wilhelm 1967). Further, local causes of pain apart from acute and chronic injury of the shoulder region and relatively rare pressure damage of the suprascapular nerve are internal diseases such as hyperuricaemia and pseudogout. Distant causes of pain such as Paget-von Schroetter syndrome, pulmonary tuberculosis, apoplectic insult and primarily myocardial infarction only lead to pain projection into the shoulder area and the arm. Distant pain can also be caused by subphrenic abscess and gall bladder, pancreatic and gastroduodenal diseases.

As diagnostic possibilities as well as conservative and surgical treatment of local causes of shoulder pain nowadays are excellent and successful, extensive denervation is not necessary in these cases. Thus, the denervation method by Nyakas and Kiss (1955) cutting only the posterior caudal articular nerve of the suprascapular and the axillar nerve in combination of an incision of the axillar recessus is only of historic interest.

On the contrary, in resistant severe pain radiation into the coracoid region, the shoulder and the AC joint, a partial denervation can be recommended. This is also true for the temporary pain elimination by blocking the entire shoulder innervation.

4.2   Surgically Relevant Anatomy and Physiology

A short synopsis concerning the shoulder innervation will be given; as in many relevant textbooks and atlases, a presentation of the articular nerves at the upper extremity is still missing. For more detailed information, I refer to the monograph by Rüdinger (1857) and the works of Gardner (1948) and see Ref. Wilhelm (1958, 1963, 1972), as well as to presentations of von Lanz and Wachsmuth (1959) and by Braus and Elze (1960).

Branches of the suprascapular nerve innervate the *extension side of the shoulder joint* (Fig. 4.1). The upper, middle and lower articular nerves innervate the scapulohumeral joint capsule extramuscularly. The cranial articular branch of the suprascapular nerve also innervates the back side of the coracoid, finally reaching the acromioclavicular joint (AC joint). Intramuscularly, two further articular nerves

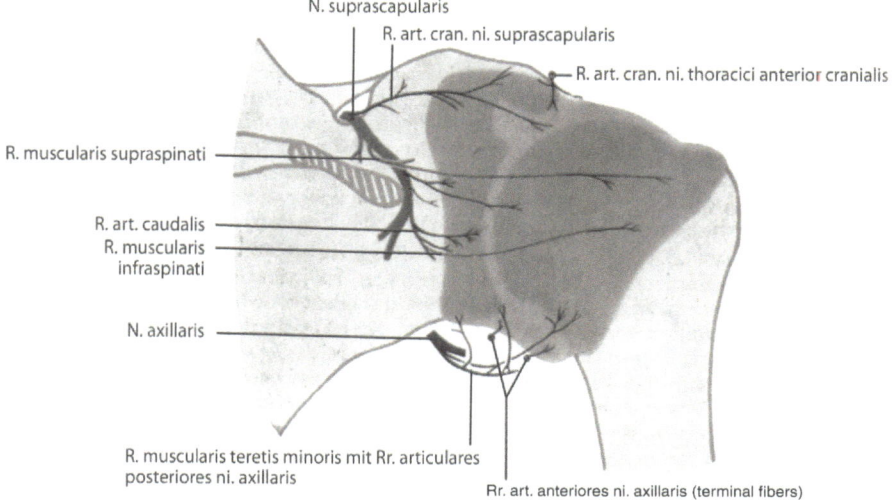

N. suprascapularis

R. art. cran. ni. suprascapularis

R. art. cran. ni. thoracici anterior cranialis

R. muscularis supraspinati

R. art. caudalis
R. muscularis
infraspinati

N. axillaris

R. muscularis teretis minoris mit Rr. articulares
posteriores ni. axillaris

Rr. art. anteriores ni. axillaris (terminal fibers)

Fig. 4.1 Posterior innervation of the shoulder joint. (From Wilhelm 1972)

come from the muscular branch of the supraspinatus and infraspinatus nerve, reaching the articular capsule at the insertion area of the muscles mentioned before. Caudally, the articular branches of the axillar nerve and the ramifications of its anterior articular branches follow at the lateral axillar hiatus.

The *shoulder joint is innervated on the flexion side* by intramuscular articular nerves in a deep layer, coming from 4 muscular branches of the subscapular nerves (Fig. 4.2). The most cranial branch also innervates the subcoracoid bursa; the remaining muscular branches end as articular fibres. The axillar recessus caudally is innervated by articular fibres of the axillar nerve before it enters the axillar gap. The most lateral articular fibres innervate the humeral capsule and the lesser tuberosity of the humerus. Figure 4.2 also shows a strikingly long subdeltoidal intertubercular branch of the axillar nerve, not only innervating the AC joint but also the major tuberosity of the humerus (Figs. 4.2 and 4.3).

An acromioclavicular articular branch is found in cranial direction in the superficial layer (Fig. 4.4), that is, in the extramuscular site, branching from the cranial anterior thoracic nerve. It runs over the coracoid process laterally, innervating it at its front and upper side and finally innervating the subacromial bursa and the AC joint. Shortly before the anterior cranial thoracic nerve enters the major pectoral muscle, a stronger nerve branch develops, running directly below the coracoid to the front rim of the deltoid muscle then branching below this muscle as variety of an intertubercular branch of the axillar nerve at the intertubercular synovial vagina (Fig. 4.4). This is normally innervated by a quite short branch of the axillar nerve up to the articular capsule (Fig. 4.5).

A branch of the caudal anterior thoracic nerve (Fig.4.4) or the musculocutaneous nerve (Fig. 4.5) innervates the subcoracoidal capsule section. Sympathetic fibres run together with this articular branch, coming from the cranial pole of the stellate

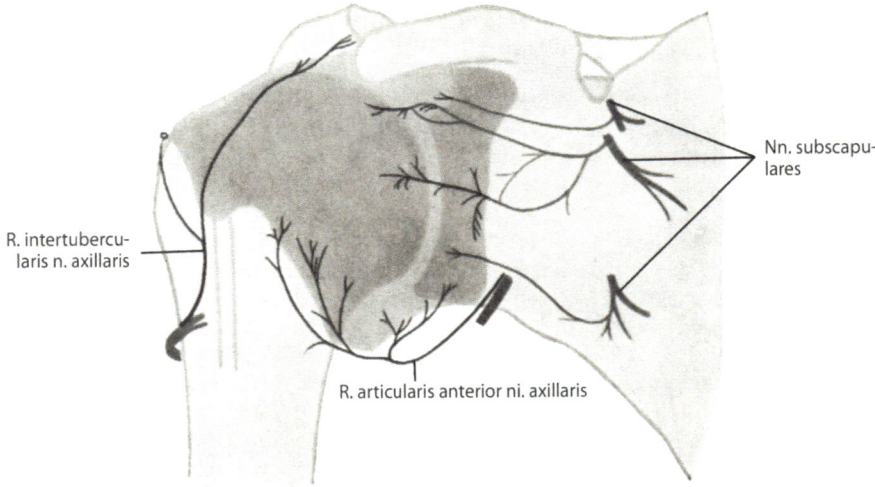

Fig. 4.2 Anterior innervation of the shoulder joint, deep layer. (From Wilhelm 1972)

Fig. 4.3 Anatomic specimen: atypical course of the axillar nerve intertubercular branch, also innervating the AC joint. (From Wilhelm 1963)

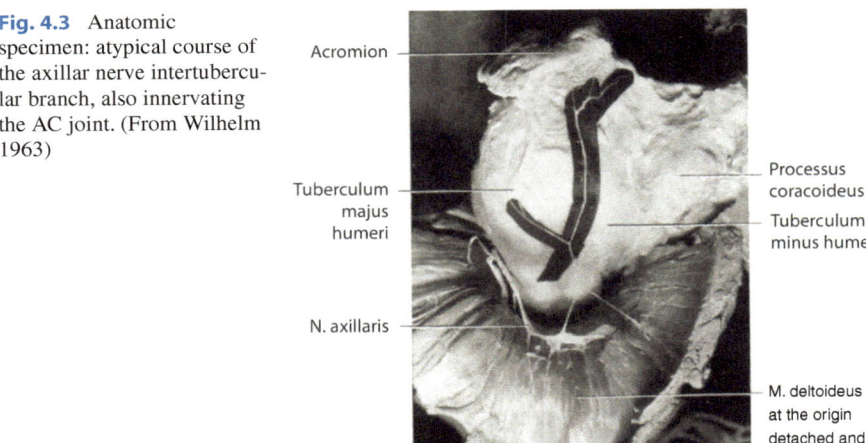

ganglion, running to the back side of the subclavian artery and continuing distally in the adventitia of this vessel, permanently providing delicate fibres. One of them runs to the origin of the thoracoacromial artery from the axillar artery, finally connecting here with the articular branch of the caudal anterior thoracic nerve. Both structures run below the lateral fascicle of the brachial plexus and then move on to the front area of the subscapular muscle together with a small capsule vessel of the thoracoacromial artery towards the coracoid. Underneath, nerves and vessels enter the scapular capsule and the subcoracoid bursa, where a fine nerve strand also innervates the lower side of the coracoid and the coracoacromial ligament (Fig. 4.4).

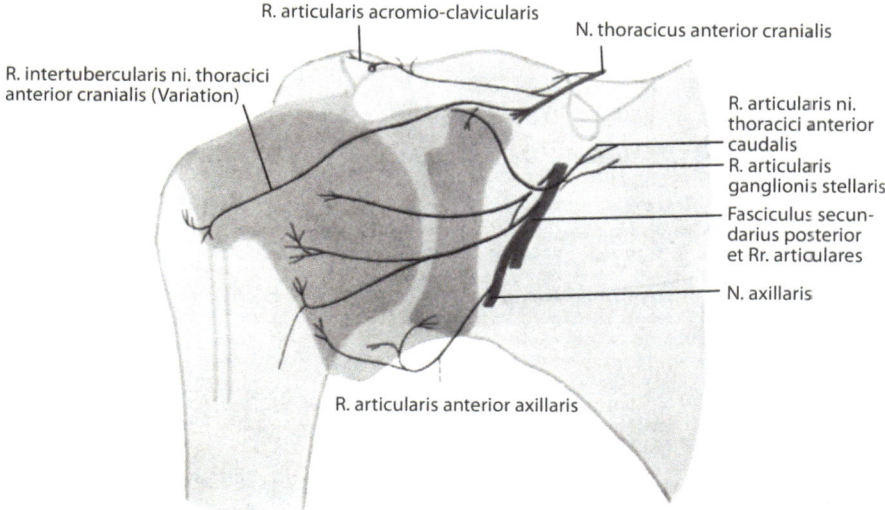

Fig. 4.4 Anterior innervation of the shoulder joint, superficial layer. (From Wilhelm 1972)

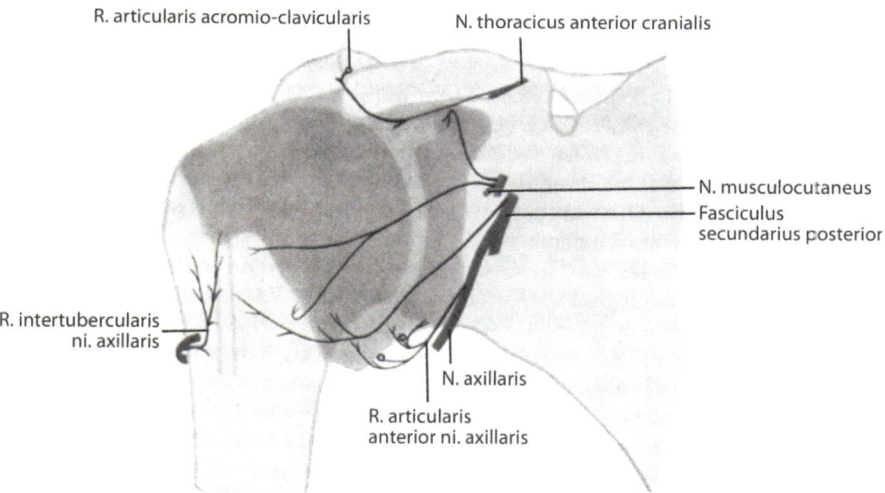

Fig. 4.5 Anterior innervation of the shoulder joint with regular course of axillar nerve intertubercular branch. (From Wilhelm 1972)

In further distal direction, two articular branches arise from the posterior fascicle, running in a slight bow over the subscapular muscle towards the minor humeral tuberculum. The lowest branch can take over a part of the axillar nerve innervation area shown in Fig. 4.2, also originating from the posterior fascicle.

4.3   Epidemiology

Pain at the anterior upper quadrant of the shoulder joint region is not rare. Basically, these complaints are caused by a *so-called coracoiditis*. These testimonials, however, do not suffice for an objective, statistical evaluation of the incidence rate. There is an indirect possibility in examining the patient population of TOS and SD. A so-called coracoiditis develops in 71 % of 100 TOS patients surgically treated. In Sudeck's dystrophy, the improvement rate accounts to 70 % of 20 patients; cf. postoperative results (Tables 5.10 and 5.11).

In so-called coracoiditis, we consequently have a projection of pain, just as in "epicondylitis".

4.4   Etiology and Pathogenesis

As already mentioned initially (cf. Sect. 4.1), partial denervation is mainly useful in treatment of resistant severe pain radiation into the coracoid and acromial region (Table 4.1), basically being accomplished via the acromioclavicular articular branch of the cranial anterior thoracic nerve and articular branches of the stellate ganglion in connection with a branch of the caudal anterior thoracic nerve (Fig. 4.4).

Pain demanding surgical treatment is based on foramen stenosis, the therapy of which is not discussed here, and especially TOS and the difficultly distinguishable early manifestations of this syndrome, also Sudeck's dystrophy (CRPS I), with a symptom complex showing striking parallels to TOS.

Pain at the AC joint and the acromion is mainly caused by arthrotic and arthritic processes, by subacromial impingement syndrome, injury of the rotator cuff and by calcificating tendinosis as well as by negative surgical results (Idelberger 1982, Tackmann et al. 1989, Wiedemann et al. 2007).

Table 4.1   Thoracic outlet syndrome (1982–1987): findings at the shoulder girdle

Preoperative findings		Postoperative results			
$N_p = 92$ – follow-up – $N_{op} = 100$		Excellent	Good	Fair	Unchanged
Occipital pain	28 →	18	2	3	5
Upper cervical syndrome	44 →	28	4	6	6
Lower cervical syndrome	72 →	50	4	10	8
Trapezius muscle	83 →	49	7	15	12
Brachial plexus	92 →	64	10	7	11
Supraspinous fossa	34 →	22	1	7	4
Infraspinous fossa	31 →	19	2	7	3
Accessory nerve	22 →	8	1	7	6
Coracoid process	71 →	46	7	8	10
Acromion	31 →	13	4	8	6
Greater tuberosity of the humerus	29 →	16	1	4	8
Deltoid insertion	48 →	37	4	4	3
Total	585 = 100 %	370 = 63.3 %	47 = 8 %	86 = 14.7 %	82 = 14 %

Modified according to Wilhelm (1997a, b), with kind permission from Thieme

Shoulder pain requiring elimination in pre- and postoperative treatment is mainly caused by primary shoulder stiffness, also called adhesive capsulitis or *frozen shoulder*, resulting in a secondary shoulder stiffness, seen postoperatively after injury and surgery of the shoulder-arm region. The so-called periarthritic attack is a further essential cause of pain, occurring in tendinosis calcarea, being diagnosed by limited areas of calcification at the rotator cuff with corresponding osteoporotic changes at the greater tuberosity of the humerus.

4.5 Diagnostics

Besides pain at the shoulder joint, patients *anamnestically* frequently complain of pain at the back of the head and the neck muscles and of pain upon motion of the shoulder and the head (Table 4.1). Also, rest pain is reported, increasing at night in contrast to motion pain of the shoulder, due to an intense traction stress of nerve roots by a decrease of muscle tone with segmental character of pain radiation.
- *Myokinetic impairment is found upon examination of characteristic muscles (C5: deltoid muscle, C6: biceps muscle, C7: triceps muscle), as well as in decrease of crude strength.*

The shoulder joint is mainly innervated by articular branches of the suprascapular nerves (C4-C6), the subscapular nerves (C5–/C7), the anterior thoracic nerves (C5-C8) and the axillar nerves (C5, C6).

A segmental examination is performed in order to exactly localise painful inhibitions of motion at the cervical spine; the behaviour of pain is checked in extension (improvement) and compression of the cervical spine (deterioration). X-rays of the cervical spine in two levels and in semi-diagonal position suffice for showing post-traumatic and degenerative articular changes, as well as stenoses of the intervertebral foramina. In ongoing segmental complaints, a CT or NMR should be performed immediately to rule out a luxation of an intervertebral disk, a tumour or an infectious/destructive process; a *neurological examination* then is necessary as well.

In the diagnosis of TOS, it primarily is most important to keep this syndrome in mind (Dunant 1975), especially since most of the patients already present with characteristic stress- and situation-connected complaints. Inspection should focus on an upward displacement of the scapula, relaxing the nerve-vessel strand in a *cervical rib*, as well as a shoulder girdle pushed forward, also relaxing the nerve-vessel bundle (Stöhr 2006).
- *An increase in diameter at the arm and hand together with an enlargement of the mamma at the same side, a pronounced venous pattern on the back of the hand and a visible collateral circle at the shoulder and chest are very important, possibly showing a venous impairment of the subclavian vein due to stenosis and congenital or acquired obstructions ("non-thrombotic occlusion" and Paget-von Schroetter syndrome).*

The colour of the skin, temperature and trophics of the hand are important. *Irritations of the brachial plexus at the upper thoracic outlet* sometimes can lead to a *Raynaud phenomenon* or frequently to a *Horner syndrome*. In atrophy of the inner hand muscles, a pressure damage of the lower plexus roots (C8 and Th1) is possible. Pulse control in hanging arm and pressure stress of the shoulder girdle, as well as *diverse provocation*

Table 4.2 Thoracic outlet-syndrome (1982–1987): finding at the elbow and the forearm

Preoperative findings			Postoperative results			
$N_p = 92$ – follow-up – $N_{op} = 100$			Excellent	Good	Fair	Unchanged
Radial tunnel – proximal part	8	→	4	–	2	2
Radial tunnel – intermediate part	34	→	14	4	8	8
Radial tunnel – distal part	29	→	21	1	3	4
Radial epicondylitis humeri	86	→	48	17	7	14
Interosseus neuralgia	22	→	18	–	1	3
Radial styloiditis	18	→	11	1	3	3
Ulnar epicondylitis humeri	23	→	18	1	1	3
Medial cutaneous nerve of the forearm	32	→	25	1	3	3
Ulnar styloiditis	7	→	4	–	1	2
Brachioradial insertion tendinopathy	10	→	4	1	1	4
De Quervain's diseases	11	→	7	1	1	2
Total:			280 = 100 %	174 = 62.2 %	27 = 9.6 %	31 = 11.1 % 48 = 17 %

Modified according to Wilhelm (1997a, b), with kind permission from Thieme

tests, like the carrying test (anamnesis), the abduction test (3-min fist-closure test) according to Roos (1979) and the elevation test, give first hints at an involvement of the vascular system, whereas redressment of the shoulder girdle can result in irritation of the lower plexus roots with radiation of pain into the area of the hand and the fingers.

A very diligent examination of the neck, shoulder, arm and hand area is essential. Notice multiple localisations of pain at the neck muscles, the trapezius muscle, the muscles of the scapula, the brachial plexus, the accessory nerve, the coracoid process, the acromion, the tubercula humeri and the deltoid insertions (Table 4.1). Pain to pressure and tension as well as sensibility disorders of peripheral nerves and their areas of innervation (tennis and golf elbow, styloiditis) are of special interest. Notice hand edema; tendovaginitis; pressure pain at the first intermetacarpal space, as well as of the thenar and the small finger; median compression; sensibility disorders at the superficial radial branch and the fingers; and acroparaesthesia. Measuring crude strength is important (Tables 4.2 and 4.3).

A table summarising these findings (cf. Chap. 5, Table 5.7) *facilitates the examination technique*, providing a much better survey, making the immediate tentative diagnosis of TOS possible (Tables 4.1, 4.2 and 4.3). *Test blockade of the stellate ganglion or the brachial plexus confirms this diagnosis. X-rays of the cervical spine* to rule out foramen stenosis are essential. A survey radiography of the upper thoracic aperture helps judging the site of the thoracic girdle and its connection to the first costa. *Cervical ribs and their rudiments*, broad and prominent transverse process of C7, as well as variations in shape and site of the first rib and the clavicle can be documented. CT and NMR are only rarely necessary.

Table 4.3 Thoracic outlet syndrome (1982–1987): findings at the hand

Preoperative findings		Postoperative results			
$Np=92$ – follow-up – $Nop=100$		Excellent	Good	Fair	Unchanged
Tendovaginitis—carpal channel	35 →	15	10	4	7
Median nerve compression	79 →	53	11	8	6
Intermetacarpal pain	28 →	13	4	5	6
Thenar pain	19 →	14	–	2	3
Hypothenar pain	7 →	6	–	1	–
Tendovaginitis I–V	38 →	17	3	6	12
Superficial branch of radial nerve	9 →	4	–	5	–
Sensibility disorder I–V	42 →	33	5	3	1
Hand edema	39 →	23	7	6	3
Acroparaesthesia	33 →	25	2	4	2
Impairment of strength	75 →	46	12	7	10
Total	404 = 100 %	248 = 61.4 %	54 = 13.3 %	52 = 12.9 %	50 = 12.4 %

Modified according to Wilhelm (1997a, b), with kind permission from Thieme

- *Examination of arm or hand edema requires a functional phlebography of the subclavian vein.*

This only slightly stressful examination allows an exact judgement of the subclavian vein inflow conditions. There is an increase of venous inflow pressure in stenosis, compression or even obstruction of this vein, radiologically leading to development of a *collateral circle* and even more important to a *reflux of contrast medium into the cephalic vein.*

Edema of the arm, the hand and the fingers is found as a result of this obstruction, objectified by comparative measurement of diameter and determination of hand volume by immersion test. These methods are also used in postoperative examination.

The phlebographic proof of compressive effects at the costoclavicular gap can give important hints at fibromuscular and other irritating structures.

In TOS patients in 79 (79 %) of 100 cases, *median nerve compressions* are found as a further result of chronic edema caused by congestion, completely vanishing after decompression of the subclavian vein in 53 (67.1 %) out of 79 patients and remaining slightly remarkable in 11 (13.9 %). Unchanged findings were documented in only 6 (7.6 %) patients.

- *Herewith and by corresponding histological examinations, the long quest for pathogenesis of the so-called idiopathic median compression resulting from chronic edema has been proved* (Wilhelm and Wilhelm 1985).

Stenotic sound, weak pulse and a blood pressure difference of 20 mmHg and more and also the suspicion of a *subclavian artery aneurysm* and *microembolic obstructions* of the peripheral vascular system definitely need an arteriogram. *Duplex* should always precede this invasive diagnostic measure (Rob and Standeven 1958).

If there is an indication for surgical treatment of therapy-resistant TOS, preoperatively infection parameters, ASL titre, rheumatic factors, uric acid and hepatic parameters should be determined. *Alcohol abuse* should be ruled out. Focal toxicity needs to be treated prior to surgery.

If additionally there are trophic and secretory disturbances, striking changes of skin temperature and colour and sensibility disorders at the medial cutaneous nerve of the forearm and the area of the ulnar nerve, but also in the area innervated by the median nerve, primarily always Sudeck's dystrophy (CRPS I) should be taken into account. This is also true for pain to touch, pressure, motion and relaxation, as well as in proof of allodynia and reduction of crude strength.

In order to prove this dystrophy blockades of the stellate ganglion or the brachial plexus, as well as x-rays of the hand (bone atrophy), the upper thoracic aperture and especially a *functional phlebography of the subclavian vein* in adduction and abduction of the arm in 90° have to be performed as additional examinations. Phlebography is essential in Sudeck, as it leads to important hints at the prognosis and especially at the importance of an early indication to surgery, on which the success of a curative procedure depends.

An *arteriography in Sudeck* needs to be delivered only in the cases mentioned above. *Bone scanning* of the hand *is not necessary* as this method is not specific and less dependable prognostically speaking (for further details on this subject, cf. Chap. 5).

4.6   Classification

For therapeutic reasons, pain in the shoulder region should be divided into an acute, a resistant to conservative therapy and a chronically recurrent form.

4.7   Indications and Contraindications

An indication for a partial denervation to limit intolerable pain radiations into the frontal upper quadrant, the coracoid region, is rare, as in most cases early conservative and surgical treatment of foramen stenosis and resistant thoracic outlet syndromes and especially of Sudeck's dystrophy leads to distinct improvement of pain (Tables 4.1, 4.2 and 4.3).

Also *postoperative pain* in the *region of the AC joint* after surgical procedures at the rotator cuff and after acromial plastic can be successfully treated by partial denervation focusing on the articular branch of the anterior cranial thoracic nerve.

Temporary pain relief by blocking the entire innervation of the shoulder joint is a very successful method to treat the so-called acute periarthritic pain attack. Also in the follow-up treatment of painful shoulder stiffness and adduction contraction, this method can be used as a favoured and successful measure.

Special contraindications for partial denervation are only found in specific limitation of operability due to disease or age, whereas there are no limitations to temporary pain relief.

4.8 Therapy

Treatment of diverse factors at the cervical spine is published in special literature.

An extensive presentation of the entire syndrome of thoracic outlet and thoracic inlet is found in Roos (1977, 1979), Wilhelm and Wilhelm (1985), Gruß et al. (1987), Leffert (1991), Narakas (1991), Mumenthaler et al. (1998), Bahm (2006), Millesi and Schmidhammer (2006) and Prescher and Schuster (2006).

Conservative and surgical therapy of Sudeck's dystrophy is presented in Chap. 5.

4.8.1 Technique of Partial Upper Frontal Shoulder Quadrant Denervation of the Shoulder Joint According to Wilhelm

An indication for partial denervation in the coracoid region is only given after test elimination, first only infiltrating the anterior innervation of the coracoid process and the subcoracoid space, in order to notice a possible pain radiation via the upper extramuscular articular branch of the suprascapular nerve (Fig. 4.1). Possibly, this conduction of pain can next be added by blockade of the suprascapular nerve.

Skin incision of 6–8 cm starts directly underneath the clavicle at the height of the coracoid process, following the inner rim of the deltoid muscle in distal direction. After incision of the deltoid muscle fascia lateral of the *cephalic vein,* this vessel is prepared in order to remain connected to the major pectoral muscle. Crossing vessels and orifice of cephalic vein branches have to be ligated and cut. *Branches of the cranial anterior thoracic nerve* for innervation of the deltoid muscle clavicular part need to be preserved (Figs. 4.4 and 4.5). After using a blunt hook, the deep pectoral fascia is found, the medial part of which coats the subclavian muscle and the minor pectoral muscle as clavipectoral fascia. The fascia in the middle of the deltoideopectoral triangle is called thoracoaxillar fascia; the lateral one is called thoracobrachial fascia. After snaring the cranial anterior thoracic nerve and its conjoining vessels feeding the clavicular portion of the deltoid muscle, the fascia at the frontal rim of the short bicipital head is incised longitudinally. Then the head of the upper arm is free and the fibres of the *coracoacromial ligament* ending in the lateral rim of the short bicipital head originating tendon can be resected in bow shape, resulting in a better view of the subcoracoidal space. If this should not suffice, as in muscular or obese patients, either the bicipital head tendinous portion of origin needs to be incised or even the peak of the coracoid process directly cut with a vibrating saw after prior drilling; afterwards, the common origins of the biceps and the coracobrachial muscle can be retracted in medial direction, preserving the origin of the minor pectoral muscle (Fig. 4.6).

First, the *articular branch of the cranial anterior thoracic nerve is eliminated,* penetrating the infraclavicular cribriformous plate of the deep pectoral fascia, turning in lateral direction at the subclavian muscle and then crossing the coracoid process running directly in front of the coracoclavicular ligament. At this point, the articular branch also innervates the entire ligament and the subcoracoid bursa (Fig. 4.5) apart from the coracoid itself, then running to the AC joint as acromioclavicular articular branch. Denervation is performed blindly by electric knife, cutting

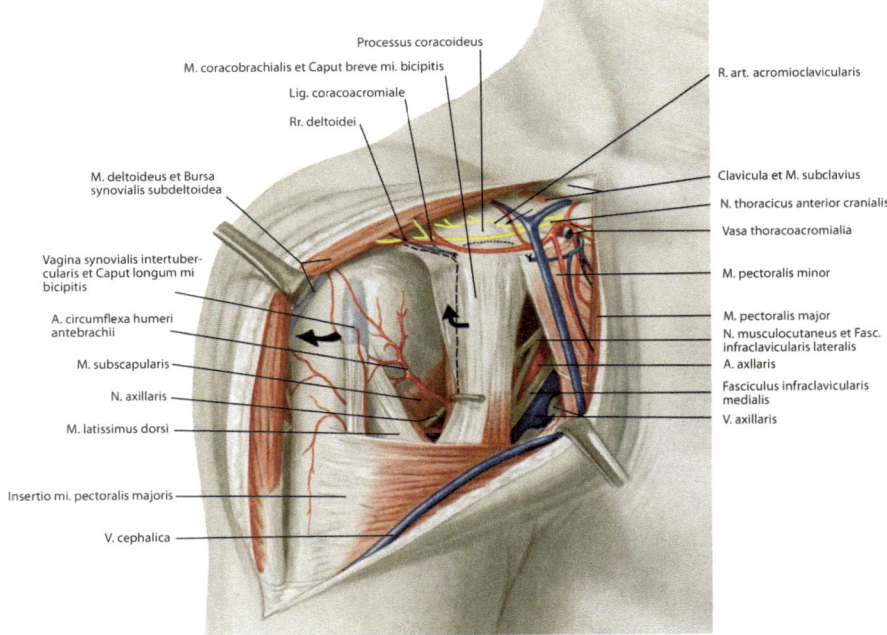

Processus coracoideus

M. coracobrachialis et Caput breve mi. bicipitis

Lig. coracoacromiale

Rr. deltoidei

R. art. acromioclavicularis

M. deltoideus et Bursa
synovialis subdeltoidea

Clavicula et M. subclavius

N. thoracicus anterior cranialis

Vasa thoracoacromialia

Vagina synovialis intertuber-
cularis et Caput longum mi
bicipitis

M. pectoralis minor

A. circumflexa humeri
antebrachii

M. pectoralis major

N. musculocutaneus et Fasc.
infraclavicularis lateralis

M. subscapularis

A. axllaris

N. axillaris

Fasciculus infraclavicularis
medialis

M. latissimus dorsi

V. axillaris

Insertio mi. pectoralis majoris

V. cephalica

Fig. 4.6 Anatomic-topographic conditions at the frontal entrance to the shoulder joint. Articular acromioclavicular branch of the cranial anterior thoracic nerve; cut off this nerve marked by *thin black arrow*. *Thin hatched line*: separation of coracoid peak above the thoracoacromial vessels. *Thick hatched line*: extent of resection of coracoacromial ligament fibres into lateral rim of short bicipital head. *Flexed thick arrow*: entrance to subcoracoid bursa and articular branch of stellate ganglion. *Slightly flexed thick arrow*: slight outer rotation of humeral head. Thoracoacromial vein at the coracoid process resected, due to optical reasons. (According to von Lanz and Wachsmuth 1959)

the tissue above the coracoid process close to the base at its anteromedial side in longitudinal direction (Fig. 4.6).

Afterwards, elimination of the *stellate ganglion articular branch*, joining a stronger articular branch of the caudal anterior thoracic nerve behind the axillar artery is performed. The common trunk of these branches then goes below the lateral fascicle and to the frontal area of the subscapular muscle to the coracoid process, underneath entering the scapular capsule, also innervating the subcoracoid synovial bursa. A delicate nerve fibre goes along the lower side of the coracoid, also innervating the coracohumeral ligament (Fig. 4.4).

After resection of the fibres coming from the coracoacromial ligament into the short bicipital head, a stump hook is used delicately, holding aside the muscle's tendon of origin and possibly also the osteotomised peak of the coracoid with the originating arm muscles. Afterwards, the lateral fascicle and the musculocutaneous nerve are localised and preserved beneath a deeper hook during preparation. A pressure damage of these structures has to be prevented absolutely. Preparation is performed along the upper rim of the subscapular muscle, also preparing the frontal side of the subcoracoid bursa in order to cut both upper intramuscular articular branches of the subscapular nerves, if necessary. The upper part of the subscapular muscle has to be loosened sharply from the humeral and scapular capsule. After finishing this preparation, the entire filling tissue remaining underneath the coracoid is excised, diligently preserving the subcoracoid bursa.

- *Also, denervation can be performed blindly below the coracoid process.*

After control of haemorrhage, suture of the incised bicipital tendon or reposition of the coracoid peak and osteosynthesis by traction screw or by two cerclage wires through the bone as well as a redon drainage, wound closure is accomplished layer by layer. After the application of a slightly compressive dressing, also including the arm, immobilisation of the arm follows in anteversion on an abduction cast with intermediate position of the forearm. Active mobilisation of the shoulder joint follows in the abduction cast.

This site also allows elimination of the remaining intramuscular *articular branches of the subscapular nerves* if necessary; it is sufficient to cut the insertion of the subscapular muscle slightly proximal to the tendinous portion of origin, like in the Eden-Hybinette procedure, sharply dissecting the proximal end to the start of the scapular capsule and afterwards reinserting it (Bauer et al. 1986).

An additional posterior approach is necessary for eliminating the cranial *extramuscular branch of the suprascapular nerve*, innervating the back side of the coracoid process and the AC joint. The incision necessary is done 2 cm above and parallel to the scapular spine by loosening the trapezius origin. The articular nerve branches out directly after passing the suprascapular notch from the main trunk running laterally outside the muscle.

As the cranial anterior thoracic nerve not only innervates the coracoid process but also the AC joint, sole resection of this nerve according to the experience of Dellon (2007) can also successfully treat persisting pain after surgery of rotator cuff defects and after acromioplasties.

4.8.2 Technique of Complete Temporary Pain Elimination at the Shoulder Joint According to Wilhelm

Blocking innervation of the shoulder joint (Fig. 4.7) should only be started after providing an i.v. access for emergency medication. This is especially applied in highly *acute periarthritic attack* in the sitting patient, where patients literally carry their painful arm into the ER. In other cases, blockade can of course also be performed in a lying position. Determination of the site of puncture in order *to block the dorsal articular branches of the suprascapular nerve* first needs palpation in the supraspinate fossa at the lengthened longitudinal axis of the coracoid process. The point for injection is found at the dorsal rim of the clavicle slightly lateral of this longitudinal axis, about one finger's breadth behind the AC joint.

After disinfection, a short needle (no. 12 or 14) is put on a 10 ml syringe and is applied vertically till it has contact to the bone. After aspiration for orientation, 3 ml of a local anaesthetic is injected slowly. In recent years, mainly *Naropin* (ropivacaine) has been used.

Fig. 4.7 Technique of complete temporary pain elimination at the shoulder joint. (From Wilhelm 1972)

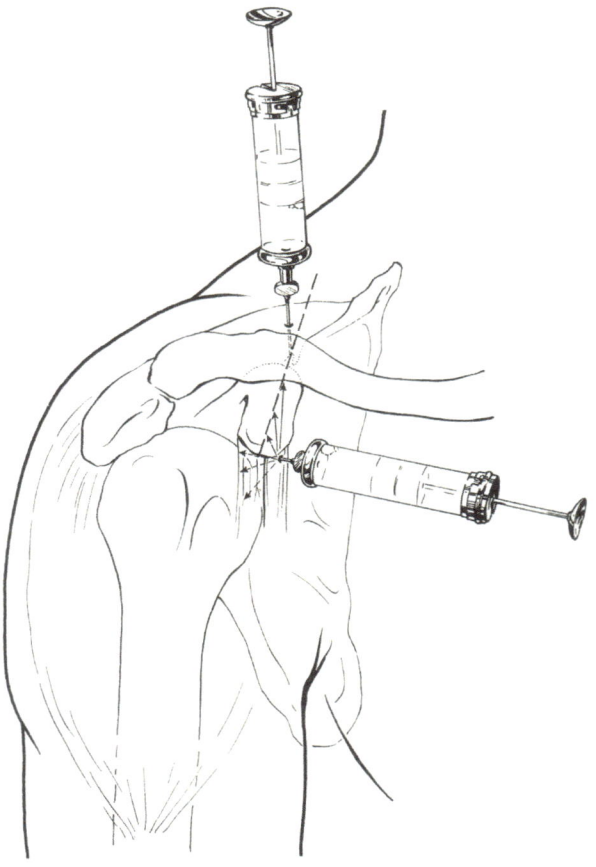

A further injection is necessary to *eliminate the anterior articular branches* (Figs. 4.2, 4.3, 4.4 and 4.5). The longitudinal axis of the coracoid process is again used for orientation. In this case, a longer needle (no. 12 or 2) is used. *Puncture is performed directly above the coracoid peak*, infiltrating the soft tissue in a fan shape up to the clavicula; 3–5 ml of local anaesthetic suffices (Figs. 4.6 and 4.7). This blockade eliminates the articular branch of the cranial anterior thoracic nerve. After injection around the coracoid process, the needle is positioned back in the subcutaneous tissue, the peak is lowered by approximately 70° in medial direction and the tissue below the coracoid is infiltrated in a fan-shaped posterolateral direction to the shoulder joint. The articular branches of the caudal anterior thoracic nerve and the stellate ganglion as well as the intramuscular branches of the subscapular nerves are eliminated. A larger amount is injected below the coracoid process in the depth between the subscapular muscle and the short bicipital head; as in this gliding layer with loose filling material there are mostly extramuscular pain leading fibres, 5–6 ml ropivacaine is needed. Finally, also the articular branches of the axillar nerve are reached by slow diffusion of the local anaesthetic (Figs. 4.2, 4.4 and 4.5).

Not earlier than 5 min after finishing the blockade, the patient is interviewed, and palpation of the areas tender on pressure before shows the success. In painful shoulder stiffness, first slight then increased active motion is performed, supported by cautious manual carrying along of the arm by the physician. After a while, degrees of abduction of 45–60° are reached, being the *first aim of treatment*, namely, the liberation of the arm out from its forced situation and the possibility of positioning it on an abduction cast. Then further mobilisation of the arm follows according to the well-known standards.

In an *acute periarthritic pain attack* and also in highly painful shoulder contraction in *thoracic outlet syndrome* or in *Sudeck's dystrophy*, 5 more minutes should pass in order to then cautiously position the arm respecting the pain tolerance in the abduction necessary in slightly flexed elbow joint and in intermediate position of the forearm on a well-padded abduction cast. Only then a shoulder x-ray for orientation as well as a local and oral anti-inflammatory medication and pain therapy should be started. Due to the muscle relaxing effect, 5 mg of diazepam should be given for the night.

This method has the *following advantages:*

1. Technically simple procedure also possible in physician's office equipped for emergencies.
2. Prevention of additional pain in local infiltration anaesthesia, for example, in the subacromial space.
3. Preservation of sufficient motion in the shoulder girdle.
4. Shortening of physiotherapeutic and postoperative duration of treatment.
5. The more difficult and complex procedures of stellate and plexus anaesthesia are not necessary as also the sympathetic innervation of the shoulder joint is interrupted.
6. Passive attempts at motion profit from a sufficient inhibition of pain, so the absence of pain reached can only be used in physiologic redressment.

Choice and dose of local anaesthetic:

A short-time local anaesthetic, such as xylocaine 1 % and scandicaine, suffices for diagnostic purpose and for application of dressings.

Longtime anaesthetic, as, for example, carbostesin, is needed for therapeutic blockade, taking into consideration the much higher toxicity. Dose in young adults over 15 years of age and in adults is 2 mg/kg body weight. In a single application with a body weight of approx. 75 kg, an entire dose of 60 ml in 0.25 % and of 30 ml in 0.5 % solution should not be exceeded.

In *severe pain situations*, such as a so-called periarthritic attack, a TOS or even in Sudeck's dystrophy, *Naropin* with an anaesthetic duration of 6–10 h has shown to be advantageous.

An exact study of the directions for use is essential in the use of carbostesin, bupivacaine and Naropin, of course. This also applies to *emergency medication,* including anticonvulsive medication, such as thiopentone sodium, dosed 1–3 mg/kg i.v. or diazepam 0.1 mg/kg i.v.

Equipment for monitoring, intubation and artificial respiration as well as resuscitation is obligatory.

4.9   Results

The first partial anterior denervation of the shoulder joint was performed at the Würzburg University Department of Surgery in 1960. At the Aschaffenburg Teaching Hospital between 1970 and 1985, only 5 patients were successfully treated surgically. A follow-up of the entire patient population from 1960 to 1985 was not possible as papers were destroyed.

Postoperative findings in surgery of TOS at the shoulder are presented in Table 4.1. The results of surgery for Sudeck are shown in Chap. 5 (Table 5.2).

The method of injection for elimination of pain was published after 3 years of trial. Success and advantages of this method were already confirmed by Gross in 1967.

4.10   Mistakes, Dangers and Complications

Dangers in partial denervation at the frontal upper quadrant of the shoulder joint region mainly consist of injury of the cephalic vein and the thoracoacromial artery as well as pressure damage of the musculocutaneous nerve and the lateral infraclavicular fascicle by sudden insertion and holding of the stump hook. Apart from common complications, there can also be a postoperative thrombotic occlusion of the subclavian vein.

Temporarily blocking the suprascapular nerve presents the danger of injection into the parallel vessels if no prior aspiration was done. In infracoracoid block, there also is the danger of an accidental puncture of the axillar vessels, if the needle was not placed in posterolateral direction; the result is an intravascular injection of local anaesthetic leading to significant toxic disturbance. For prevention, frequent aspiration attempts should be made before and during application, and injection of the anaesthetic should be done very slowly in increasing dose, starting with 25 mg/min to maximum 50 mg/min, that is, 3.6 ml to 6.6 ml/min. In accidental puncture of the vessels mentioned, there is danger of bleeding, also in puncture of the axillar artery.

References

Bahm J (2006) Systematisch-kritische Betrachtung der Problematik des Thoracic outlet-Syndroms: Klinik und Therapie [Systematic- critical consideration of the thoracic-outlet-syndrome problem]. Handchir Mikrochir Plast Chir 38:56–63

Bauer R, Kerschbaumer F, Poisel S (1986) Operative Zugangswege in Orthopädie und Traumatologie [Surgical approaches in orthopaedics and traumatology]. Thieme, Stuttgart/New York, p S217

Braus H, Elze C (1960) Anatomie des Menschen [Human anatomy], Band III, 2. Aufl. Springer, Berlin/Göttingen/Heidelberg, pp S181–S184

Dellon AL (2007) Pain solutions. Lightning Source, La Vergne

Dunant JH (1975) Diagnostik des Schultergürtelsyndroms [Diagnostics of shoulder girdle syndrome]. Therap Umschau 32:361–365

Gardner E (1948) The innervation of shoulder joint. Anat Rec 102:1–4

Gross F (1967) Die Schultersteife (Frozen Shoulder]. Arztl Fortbild 17:37–40

Gruß JD, Hiemer W, Bartels D (1987) Klinik, Diagnostik und Therapie des Thoracic outlet-Syndroms [Clinic, diagnostics, and therapy of thoracic-outlet-syndrome]. VASA (Zschr Gefäßchir) 16, pp S337–S344

Idelberger K (1982) Degenerative Erkrankungen des Schultergelenkes [Degenerative diseases of the shoulder joint]. In: Witt AN, Rettig H, Schlegel KF (Hrsg) Spezielle Orthopädie – Obere Extremität, Bd VI, Teil 2 der Orthopädie in Praxis und Klinik. Thieme, Stuttgart, pp S4.1–S4.29

Leffert RD (1991) Thoracic outlet-syndrome. In: Tubiana R (Hrsg) The hand, vol IV. Saunders, Philadelphia, pp S343–S351

Millesi H, Schmidhammer R (2006) Faszienräume und Rezidiveingriffe beim Thoracic outlet-Syndrom [Fascia spaces and procedures in relapse in thoracic-outlet-syndrome]. Handchir Mikrochir Plast Chir 38:14–19

Mumenthaler M, Schliak H, Stöhr M (1998) Thoracic outlet-Syndrom (TOS). In: Läsionen peripherer Nerven und radikuläre Syndrome. Thieme, Stuttgart, pp S240–S247

Narakas AO (1991) Cervico-brachial compression. In: Tubiana R (Hrsg) The Hand, vol IV. Saunders, Philadelphia, pp S352–S389

Nyakas A, Kiss T (1955) Von Schultergelenksarthrosen stammende Schmerzen – Heilung durch Denervation [Pain from shoulder joint arthrosis- cure by Denervation]. Zbl Chir 80:955–958

Prescher A, Schuster D (2006) Die Anatomie der seitlichen Halsregion mit besonderer Berücksichtigung des Thoracic outlet-Syndroms [Anatomy of lateral neck region with special focus on the thoracic-outlet-syndrome]. Handchir Mikrochir Plast Chir 38:6–13

Rob CHG, Standeven A (1958) Arterial occlusion complicating thoracic outlet compression syndrome. Brit Med J 2:709–712

Roos DB (1977) Transaxillary extrapleural thoracic sympathectomy. In: Surgical techniques illustrated, vol 2. Little, Braun and Co, Boston

Roos DB (1979) New concepts of thoracic outlet syndrome that explain etiology, symptoms, diagnosis and treatment. VASC Surg 13:113–121

Rüdinger N (1857) Die Gelenknerven des menschlichen Körpers [Articular nerves of the human body]. Enke, Erlangen

Stöhr R (2006) Thoracic outlet-Syndrom – Diagnostische Hinweise, Operationstechnik und Resultate [Thoracic-outlet-syndrome - diagnostic hints, surgical technique, and results]. Handchir Mikrochir Plast Chir 38:46–50

Tackmann W, Richter HP, Stöhr M (1989) Kompressionssyndrome peripherer Nerven [Compression syndromes of peripheral nerves]. Springer, Berlin/Heidelberg, pp S106–S123

von Lanz T, Wachsmuth W (1959) Praktische Anatomie [Practical anatomy], Bd I, Teil 3. Springer, Berlin/Heidelberg

Wachsmuth W, Wilhelm A (1967) Zur Ätiologie, Diagnose und Behandlung unklarer Schmerzzustände an der Handwurzel [Etiology, diagnosis, and treatment of obscure pain syndromes at the wrist]. Mschr Unfallheilk 70:89–110

Wiedemann E, Rolf O, Gohlke F (2007) Verletzungen und degenerative Erkrankungen der Schulter [Injuries and degenerative diseases of the shoulder]. In: Wirth CJ, Mutschler W (Hrsg) Praxis der Orthopädie und Unfallchirurgie. Thieme, Stuttgart/New York, pp S817–S840

Wilhelm A (1958) Die Innervation der Gelenke der oberen Extremität [Joint Innervation of the Upper Extremity]. Z Anat Entwickl Gesch 120:331–371

Wilhelm A (1963) Die gezielte Schmerzausschaltung am Schultergelenk und ihre anatomischen Grundlagen [Aimed pain elimination at the shoulder joint and its anatomical basis]. Langenbeck's Arch Klin Chir 302:799–809

Wilhelm A (1972) Die gezielte Schmerzausschaltung am Schultergelenk [Aimed pain elimination at the shoulder joint]. In: Wachsmuth W, Wilhelm A (eds) Die Operationen an der Hand, Bd X. Springer, Berlin/Heidelberg, pp S50–S54

Wilhelm A (1997a) Stenosis of the subclavian vein. An unknown cause of resistant reflex sympathetic dystrophy. Hand Clin 13:387–411

Wilhelm A (1997b) Operative Behandlung der therapieresistenten Sudeck'schen Dystrophie durch transaxilläre Dekompression des Nervengefäßstranges und Sympathektomie. Zur Pathogenese des M. Sudeck [Surgical treatment of therapy resistant Sudeck´s dystrophy by transaxillary decompression of nerve- vessel- bundle and sympathectomy. Handchir Mikrochir Plast Chir 29:60–72

Wilhelm A, Wilhelm F (1985) Das Thoracic outlet-Syndrom und seine Bedeutung für die Chirurgie der Hand [The thoracic-outlet-syndrome and its significance for hand surgery]. Handchir 17:173–187

Controversial Pain Syndrome of M. Sudeck (RSD, CRPS I): Pathogenesis and Surgical Treatment of Resistant Cases

5

Contents

5.1	Introduction	101
5.2	Surgically Relevant Anatomy and Physiology	102
5.3	Epidemiology	106
5.4	Aetiology and Pathogenesis	108
5.5	Diagnostics	111
5.5.1	Tabular Documentation of Pathologic Findings at the Upper Extremity	111
5.5.2	Phlebography of Subclavian Vein	117
5.5.3	Arteriography of Subclavian Artery	122
5.5.4	Brachial Plexus and Intraoperative Findings	124
5.5.5	Differential Diagnosis	124
5.6	Classification	125
5.7	Indications and Contraindications	125
5.8	Surgical Treatment of Resistant Cases	126
5.8.1	History	126
5.8.2	Informed Patient Consent	127
5.8.3	Instruments	128
5.8.4	Surgical Technique of Transaxillary Decompression of Neurovascular Bundle and Extrapleural Resection of Upper Sympathetic Trunk, Respectively, Neurotomy of Communicating Branches Running Towards the Lower Plexus Roots	129
5.9	Postoperative Treatment	134
5.10	Results	138
5.11	Pain Inhibitory Function of Dorsal Horn Synapsis System	143
5.12	Mistakes, Dangers and Complications	147
References		147

5.1 Introduction

Posttraumatic dystrophy was first completely described by Sudeck in 1900 and 1902. Apart from four cardinal symptoms, he also mentions secondary symptoms and the term "reflectory trophoneurosis". This pain syndrome thus can justly be called Sudeck's dystrophy or Sudeck's disease, a term only rarely found in Anglo-American

A. Wilhelm, *Controversial Pain Syndromes of the Arm*,
DOI 10.1007/978-3-642-54513-9_5, © Springer-Verlag Berlin Heidelberg 2015

literature. In French literature it has been called "algodystrophie reflexe" (Bircher 1981) and in English literature "reflex sympathetic dystrophy" (RSD, Lankford 1993), whereas the internationally acknowledged term "reflex regional pain syndrome" (CRPS I) is used. In contrast, the causalgia first described by Mitchel et al. (1864) has since been called CRPS II. Nevertheless, we should not forget the names of both distinguished and prominent authors, and we should further on use them.

Until today, Sudeck's dystrophy has been regarded as a "mysterious" disease. Aetiologically quite completely analysed in the meantime, but in pathogenetical aspect it was only agreed upon the fact the disease is based on a vasomotoric dysfunction of the sympathetic nerve system (Leriche 1923; Lankford 1993).

Though local results of this dystrophy already received extensive scientific and clinical examination, still the question remains why identical outer conditions lead to the disease in one patient, at the same time sparing another patient. Only a so-called individual predisposition for Sudeck's dystrophy has been found in literature as hypothesis for this striking fact (Blumensaat 1956) or the "incalculable phenomenon" as postulated by Hackethal (1958).

An elevated sympathetic activity prior to the start of dystrophy can be evaluated as a predisposing factor, found in diligent examination of the upper extremity, especially in diverse pain localizations, trigger points and disturbances of sensibility. A satisfactory solution of these problems is, however, not given. Searching for further predisposing factors, parallels to the symptoms of a "thoracic outlet syndrome" (TOS) were found. Thus, the application of diagnostic tools used for TOS made sense in Sudeck's dystrophy as well. This is especially true for the functional phlebography of the subclavian vein, since both diseases are characterised by edema, among others (Wilhelm and Wilhelm 1985).

The phlebographic examinations performed since the beginning of 1982 showed a more or less dominant impairment of venous run-off in Sudeck's dystrophy, seen even more clearly the higher the arterial run-in is in the upper extremity Wilhelm and Wilhelm 1985.

- *This disturbance leads to an impairment of the venous backflow, mainly causing edema in TOS and in Sudeck's dystrophy, also after injury and surgical procedures. Pathogenesis of idiopathic median nerve compression is also based on edema, as histologically shown in the meantime, and also proved by postoperative results* (Wilhelm and Wilhelm 1985; Fig. 5.1).

Improvement rates in median compression after surgical treatment of TOS are 81 % (64 out of 79 cases (Chap. 5, Table 5.2).

Phlebographic proof of subclavian vein stenosis also found in *Sudeck's dystrophy is the "second key"* (Lankford 1993) being searched for all over the world for solution of this disease.

5.2   Surgically Relevant Anatomy and Physiology

Transaxillary decompression of the nerve-vessel bundle originally developed and described by Roos (1977) for the treatment of thoracic outlet syndrome is also used for the treatment of therapy-resistant dystrophy with the precondition of exact knowledge about the anatomy of the axillary region.

Fig. 5.1 Schematic presentation of aetiology and pathogenesis of median compression caused by edema (ideopathic). (From Wilhelm and Wilhelm 1985, with kind permission from Thieme)

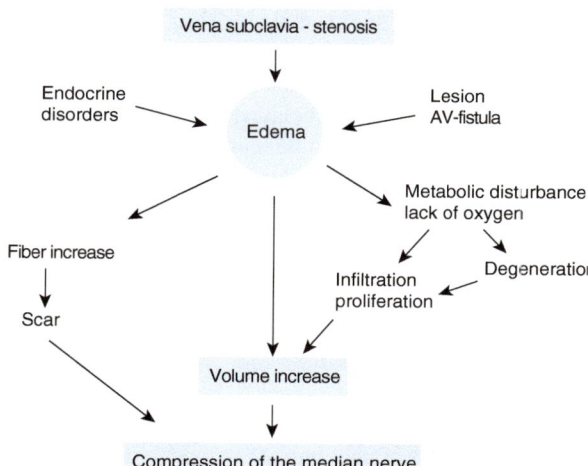

According to von Lanz and Wachsmuth (1959), the axillary region in an abducted arm is a four-sided pyramid with its peak behind the middle of the clavicle. The shape of this pyramid changes depending on arm position. Its floor is the axillary fascia.

Superficially the major pectoral muscle and in the depth the minor pectoral muscle and the subclavian muscle constitute the front wall of the axilla. The back wall consists of three muscles, being the subscapular, the teres major and the latissimus dorsi muscle, whereas the medial wall of the pyramid consists of the lateral serratus muscle and the convex thoracic wall below. The lateral wall is the most narrow one, only developed at the base of the pyramid. The inner side is bordered by the coracobrachial muscle, the short head of the biceps muscle, as well as the humerus.

Muscles of the front and the back wall meet at the shoulder joint; thus, the pyramid at its peak is only bordered on three sides.

If the axillary fascia is cut at the 3rd costa in vertical direction, you find the *thoracoepigastric vein and its lymphatic vessels* in the middle part of the superficial axillary filling tissue layer and medially the lateral thoracic vessels. *The thoracodorsal nerve and its vessels* are found in a deeper layer at the upper rim of the dorsal latissimus muscle. In further preparation, you reach the lateral serratus muscle in the depth and above it laterally and vertically the *long thoracic nerve*.

The intercostobrachial nerve with its fibres branching from the intercostal nerve II and III (Fig. 5.25) is found in further proximal direction at the height of the middle axillary line.

The *superior thoracic vessels* are situated in further laterocranial direction, running into the first intercostal space and coming from the lower side of the subclavian vessels. After ligature and cutting of the superior thoracic vessels and extension of the arm in abduction, you see the first costa and above it the vessels leading to the arm as well as the brachial plexus. In the anterior area of this region, internationally called *thoracic outlet*, there is a strikingly tendinous origin of the *subclavian muscle* from the bone-cartilage border of the 1st costa, grasping the *subclavian vein* in bow shape at the lower and frontal side (Fig. 5.25). This muscle inserts at the lower side of the clavicula, and it can *compress* the subclavian vein also from cranial direction if developed strongly. Behind the subclavian vein the *anterior scalene muscle* is situated. It divides the subclavian vein from the subclavian artery. The originating portion of this muscle can be tendinous at the back rim but also at the entire width, in functional stress of the shoulder joint leading to an *irritation of the subclavian artery and the sympathetic fibres running peripherally*, coming from the stellate ganglion (Figs. 5.25 and 5.27).

Usually the *brachial plexus* (C4–Th 1) runs next to the subclavian artery in the gap bordered by the anterior and medius scalene muscles, called hiatus scalenorum. Division of both structures is *frequently accomplished by the minor scalene muscle or its ligamentary rudiment.* These structures can also lead to irritation (Fig. 5.25).

The *minor scalene muscle* normally arises from the transverse process of the 7th cervical vertebra connecting at the inner side of the 1st costa. Its origin can additionally reach up to the height of the 5th vertebra. The relatively broad muscle in this case sometimes connects with the cupula pleurae as the so-called scalenopleural muscle (Fig. 5.2).

Retaining ligaments coming from the side of the cervical vertebra can also start behind the subclavian artery. Sometimes they radiate in front of the subclavian artery as *pleurovertebral ligament*, hindering the vessel. Most frequent special cases of the *minor scalene muscle and the pleurovertebral ligament are compiled in Fig. 5.2.*

The anterior scalene muscle comes from the 3rd to the 6th, the median scalene muscle even from the 2nd to the 7th transverse process. Behind the median scalene muscle, there is the *posterior scalene muscle* arising from the transverse processes of the 4th–6th cervical vertebrae and in contrast to the muscles mentioned before only connecting to the 2nd costa.

In preoperative presentation of the anterior scalene muscle according to von Lanz and Wachsmuth (1955), seven varieties are found:

1. The muscle can be missing altogether, also together with both other scalene muscles.
2. The muscle can connect to the 1st costa behind the subclavian artery melted with the median scalene muscle.
3. Even if there is a scalene hiatus, the subclavian artery can perforate and split the muscle.
4. The muscle can also originate from long neck costae.
5. The anterior scalene muscle can exchange its bundle of origin with the median scalene muscle.
6. The origins can be tightly connected to the intertransverse muscles.
7. If the minor scalene muscle is missing, it might be replaced by a band-like structure coming from the costotransversal process of the 7th cervical vertebra or from the neck of the 1st costa as pleurocostal ligament, then connecting at the site of the cupula pleurae.

Most of the structures mentioned can only be seen after dissociation of the anterior and median scalene muscles from the 1st costa.

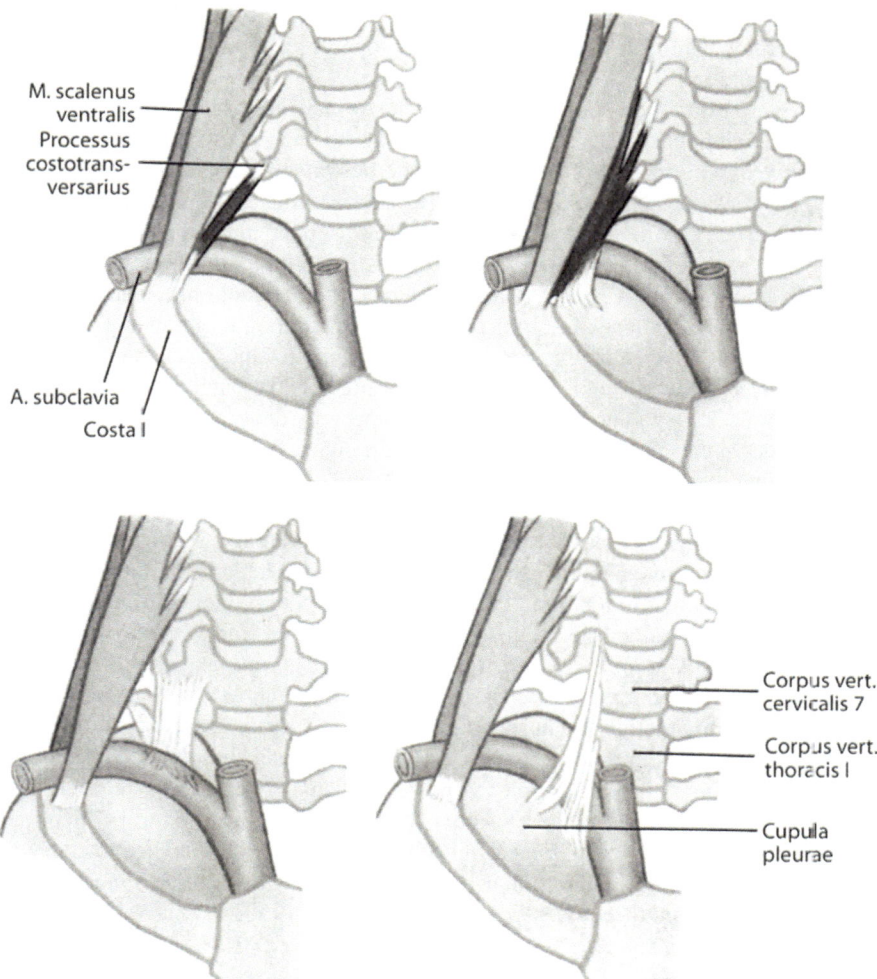

M. scalenus
ventralis
Processus
costotrans-
versarius

A. subclavia

Costa I

Corpus vert.
cervicalis 7

Corpus vert.
thoracis I

Cupula
pleurae

Fig. 5.2 Varieties of scalenus minimus muscle and pleurovertebral ligament. (From von Lanz and Wachsmuth 1955)

Resection of the 1st costa is necessary in order to exactly judge the conditions at the cupula pleurae, simultaneously decompressing the nerve-vessel bundle. Here the parietal pleura is additionally protected by a loose membrane from the chest wall (so-called endothoracic fascia). This fascia is also additionally secured at the cupula pleurae by a suprapleural membrane, also called *Sibson fascia*.

If developed strongly, this membrane can lead to compression of the subclavian vein in posterior-anterior direction (Fig. 5.10) and, in enclosure of the internal thoracic vessels and the phrenic nerve, even lead to a stripe-shaped stenosis of the vessel (Fig. 5.12)

The topographic anatomic findings at the back wall of the subclavian vein and the structures behind it in the upper thoracic opening can only be seen after blunt loosening and pushing down the cupula pleurae.

The phrenic nerve (C3–5) runs along the frontal area of the anterior scalene muscle (leading muscle!), crossing the origin of the internal thoracic artery and then normally running medial of this vessel at the back part of the subclavian vein into the upper thoracic aperture. There are diverse variations to be noticed. Rarely the phrenic nerve can run along the front side of the subclavian vein, or it can enclose this vessel with anterior and posterior portions. Also it can perforate the vein centrally in a button hole. Very rarely there is an additional (side) phrenic nerve coming from C8 and Th1, connecting with the main stem of the phrenic nerve below this vessel. A side phrenic nerve is found in 10 % (von Lanz and Wachsmuth 1955).

There is an open view of the upper thoracic vertebra, after having taken into account the anatomic topographic conditions of the upper thoracic aperture and loosening pushing down the cupula pleurae until below the subclavian vein. After removing the filling tissue, there is the upper sympathetic thoracic bundle with its communicating branches and ganglia, stored in the lamellae of the prevertebral fascia.

Regularly there is a caudal cervical ganglion, frequently melted with the first thoracic ganglion into a relatively large irregular starry shaped structure, the *stellate ganglion*. It is found in a dimple between the transverse process of the 7th cervical vertebra and the neck of the 1st costa (Fig. 5.3, von Lanz and Wachsmuth 1959).

It is easier to first look for the 3rd or 2nd thoracic ganglion and put it in a rubber band or cut and then dissect it further in cranial direction. In a stellate ganglion not only the communicating branches but also the fibres of the inferior cardiac nerves should be dissected in order to preserve them if there is a sympathetic resection by resection of the stellate ganglion inferior part. This is not always possible in an isolated ganglion T1 (Fig. 5.3). In order to be complete, it needs to be mentioned that the stellate ganglion provides a quite strong branch to the subclavian artery surrounding it in peripheral direction in plexus shape. A stronger branch innervates the coracoid region and the subcoracoid space (Wilhelm 1958; 1972).

5.3   Epidemiology

CRPS I is most frequently found after surgical treatment and after trauma of the upper extremity, independent of its severity. As already known, an abnormal sympathetic activity is the cause (Leriche 1923).

As *second key* giving a clue for pathogenesis, we found a disturbance of venous flow at the subclavian vein, also shown in phlebography (cf. 5.4, Figs. 5.5, 5.9, 5.10, 5.11, 5.12, 5.13, 5.14, 5.15, 5.16, 5.17, 5.18 and 5.19). Venous stenosis without simultaneous sympathetic hyperactivity only leads to a hand-finger syndrome (Figs. 5.5 and 5.6).

The incidence of this dystrophy is hard to judge as mainly minor and milder atypical forms are not immediately recognised and diagnosed.

Further on edema, damage by immobilisation and also artefacts are falsely interpreted as dystrophy.

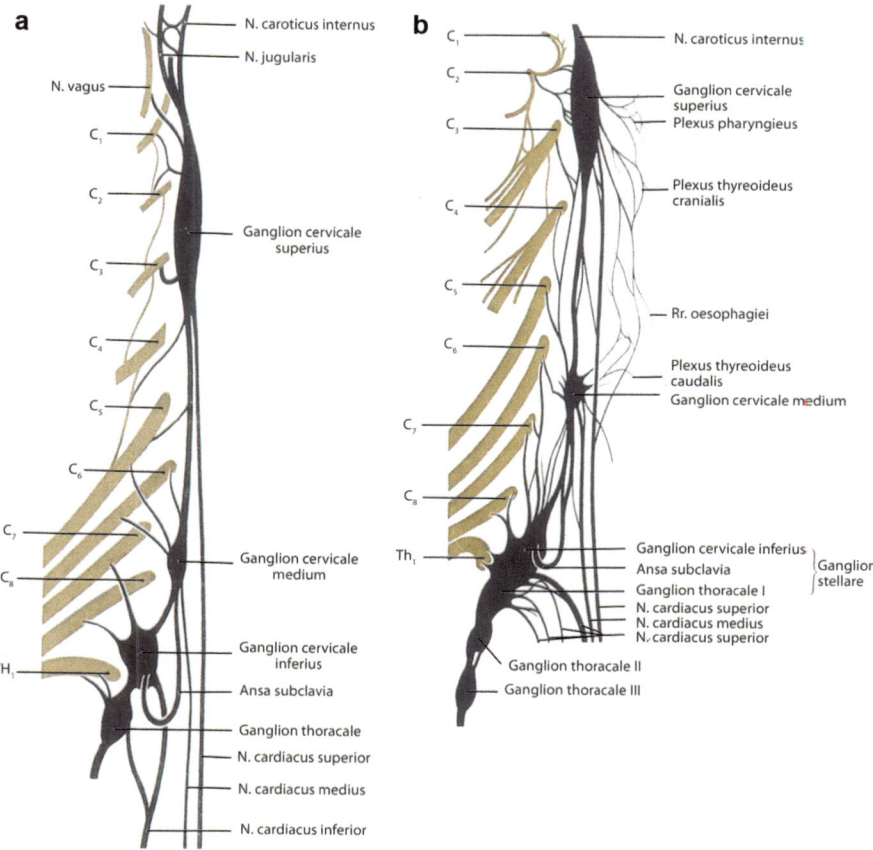

Fig. 5.3 (**a**) Inferior cervical and thoracic ganglion not melted, (**b**) inferior cervical ganglion and thoracic ganglion melted into stellate ganglion. (From von Lanz and Wachsmuth 1955)

In literature the risk of suffering from CRPS I is estimated to range between 0.05 and 5 % (according to Bär et al. 2002).

Algodystrophy is far more frequently found in females, the dominant arm being affected slightly more. This dystrophy can also occur bilaterally in rare cases. The existence of a bilateral subclavian vein stenosis is responsible. In severe dystrophy there might also be slighter symptoms.

A striking increase of this dystrophy in typical radial fracture has been analysed by now. There is a further pathogenetic factor being the compression of the deep radial branch by the supinator arcade under tension in immobilisation in forearm pronation (Werner 1979).

Family history of frequent CRPS I has also been solved pathogenetically. The cause is a disturbance of sympathetic function and a stenosis of the subclavian vein with impairment of venous flow. These factors are inheritable, whereas trauma only triggers CRPS I.

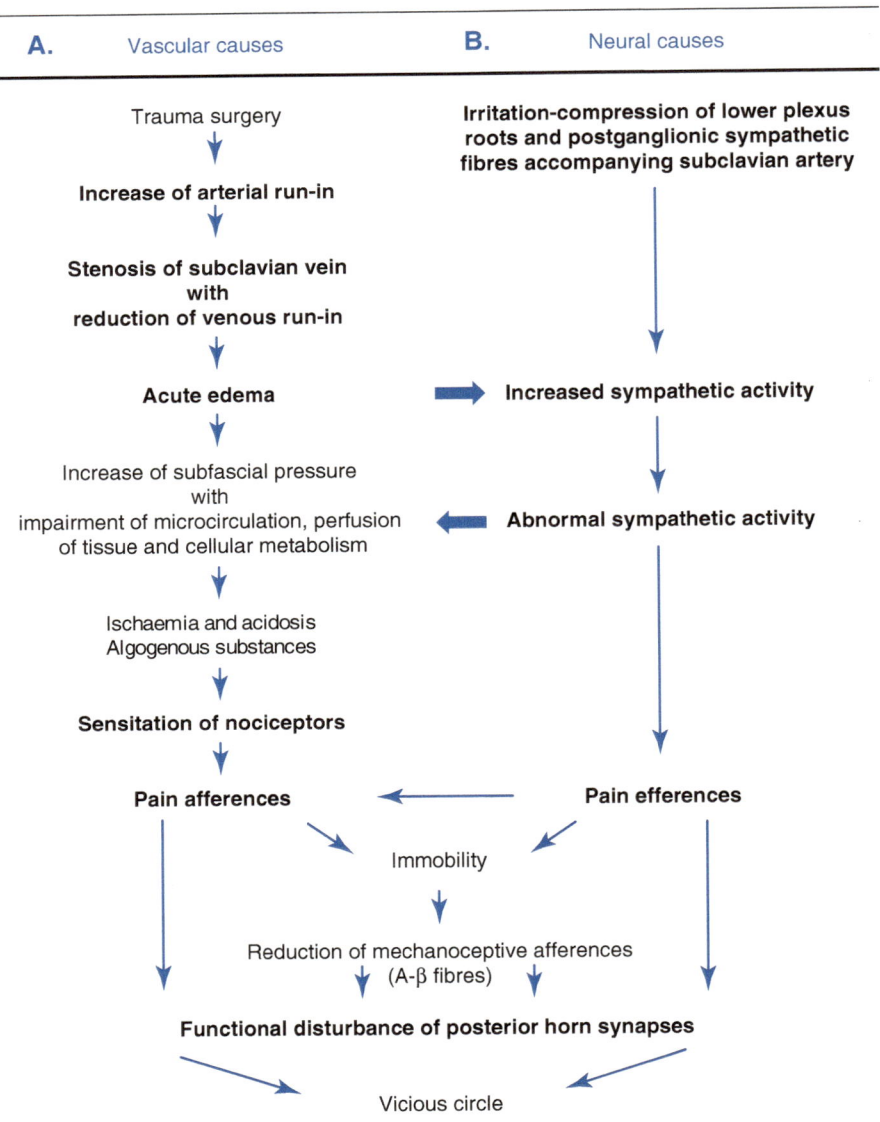

A.   Vascular causes   **B.**   Neural causes

Trauma surgery

Increase of arterial run-in

Stenosis of subclavian vein
with
reduction of venous run-in

Acute edema

Increase of subfascial pressure
with
impairment of microcirculation, perfusion
of tissue and cellular metabolism

Ischaemia and acidosis
Algogenous substances

Sensitation of nociceptors

Pain afferences

Irritation-compression of lower plexus
roots and postganglionic sympathetic
fibres accompanying subclavian artery

Increased sympathetic activity

Abnormal sympathetic activity

Pain efferences

Immobility

Reduction of mechanoceptive afferences
(A-β fibres)

Functional disturbance of posterior horn synapses

Vicious circle

Fig. 5.4 Pathogenesis of CRPS I. (From Wilhelm 1997b, with kind permission from Thieme)

5.4   Aetiology and Pathogenesis

Aetiology is still seen as an unsolved problem, even though the significance of an *elevated sympathetic tonus* has been known as a neural cause since Leriche (1923). The same is true for triggering and favouring factors.

Fig. 5.5 Functional phlebography of left subclavian vein with 80 % stenosis (*white arrow*) and collateral blood flow (*bended arrow*) and reflux into the cephalic vein (*VC, black arrow*). *BVS* valvular bulb of subclavian vein. (From Wilhelm and Englert 1989, with kind permission from Thieme)

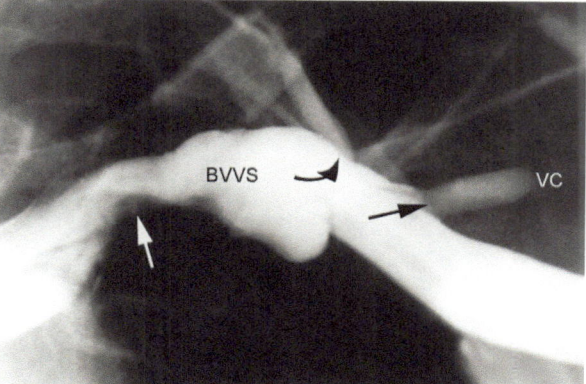

Fig. 5.6 Hand edema due to stenosis of subclavian vein after surgery for Dupuytren contraction. (From Wilhelm and Englert 1989, with kind permission from Thieme)

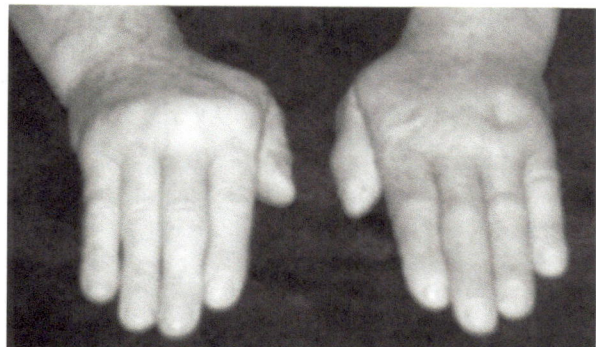

Strikingly the development of dystrophy does not depend on the severity of trauma; on the contrary, this disease often develops after minor injuries, such as contusions of the hand or shoulder region or contortions, the delayed course until the complete expression of dystrophy often lasting 1–3 months, thus diagnostically judged only sophistically in the initial phase. First increase of edema and impairment of hand function are diagnosed (Table 5.1).

The frequency of CRPS I is striking in radial fracture, where mainly pressure damage by plaster cast is accused. Remember the fact that in the immobilisation of fracture in pronation according to findings concerning pathogenesis of tennis elbow, the deep branch of the radial nerve is under permanent pressure by the supinator arcade, being 40–50 mmHg according to the findings of Werner (1979). This pressure suffices to cut off the intraneural blood flow and the axonal flow, resulting in pain afferences.

These dystrophies also occur frequently after arthroscopy (2.3 %) of the wrist and after median decompression, in 5 %, being a milder form of reflex dystrophy. Inflammatory processes, especially at the hand, can cause dystrophy (Figs. 5.36 and 5.37). Further predisposing and triggering factors are foramen stenosis at the lower cervical spine and cervical disk prolapse. Iatrogenic causes are also paravascular

Table 5.1   CRPS I (1984–1991 and 2000–2002): cases resistant to therapy

Pat. no.	Triggering causes	Pat. no.	Triggering causes
1	Radius fracture	11	Radius fracture
2	Tennis elbow	12	Crush injury
3	Shoulder contusion	13	Fracture MC II
4	Hand contusion	14	Bowling
5	Surgery of scaphoid bone	15	Rupture extensor tendon
6	Radius fracture	16	Radius fracture
7	Palmar phlegmon	17	TE surgery, according to Hohmann
8	Fracture MC II–IV	18	TE surgery, according to Hohmann
9	Hand contusion	19	Sudoriparous abscess
10	Cut	20	r/o scaphoid bone fracture

From Wilhelm (2007)

injections of contrast media, cytostatics, other medications and the accidental injection into a nerve, for example, the median nerve. Predisposing factors in internal medicine are hemiplegia and predominantly myocardial infarction.

- *The proof of the "second key"* (Lankford 1993) *was the missing link for the solution of CRPS I pathogenesis.*

First hints were found in the beginning of the 1980s in the shape of a phlebographic proof of subclavian vein stenosis (Wilhelm and Wilhelm 1985), finally responsible as the supraordinate cause of a peripheral vascular disturbance.

- *In simplified presentation pathogenesis of Sudeck's dystrophy is essentially based on a superior vascular and neural cause (Fig. 5.4). First hints at the significance of an impairment of venous run-in for this dystrophy were already described by Sudeck in* 1931 *as a result of a femoral vein thrombosis.*

In the meantime it was detected that the primary cause of painful edema is not found at the hand, where up to now an impairment of venous run-in, caused by sympathetically regulated tightening of venules, but further proximally at the upper thoracic aperture in form of a subclavian vein stenosis. The venous run-in is already more or less impaired depending on the amount of run-off disturbance, resulting in venous stasis and then in acute edema by sudden increase in arterial run-in after trauma and surgical procedures, finally leading to an increase in subfascial pressure (Grünert 1993).

Results of edema only lead to abnormal sympathetic reaction if prior to the start of the disease the patient already had an increased sympathetic activity.

Apart from central mechanisms causes are mainly irritations and compressions of the lower plexus roots by the inner rim of the 1st costa, by fibromuscular structures as well as by the postganglion sympathetic fibres accompanying the subclavian artery.

Abnormal sympathetic activity then, due to vasoconstriction, leads to further deterioration of microcirculation, perfusion of tissue and cell metabolism already worsened by edema. The results are ischemia and acidosis, and as an effect of the algogenic agents that develop, it leads to an increase of irritability of nociceptors with consecutive increase of pain afferences.

Sudeck's dystrophy manifests as soon as the sum of pain afferences and efferences leads to an "overstress" and to immobilisation with resulting reduction of pain-inhibiting mechanoceptive afferences. A "vicious circle" results (Zimmermann and Handwerker 1984).

Now both of the most important causal factors of SD are known and can be localised and documented by phlebography and arteriography. The so-called individual predisposition for Sudeck's dystrophy (Hackethal 1958) then is primarily based on an impairment of venous run-off at the subclavian vein, resulting in a disbalance of arterial run-in and venous run-off at a simultaneously elevated sympathetic activity. In a normal sympathetic regulation of reflexes, venous stenosis under identical external conditions (surgery, trauma, etc.) only leads to an edema of the hand. Figures 5.5 and 5.6 show an example.

• *Finally Sudeck's dystrophy can be calculated by the introduction of functional phlebography, being significant not only in forensic and legal (insurance) respect.*

Taking into account the anatomic, topographic and pathophysiologic facts, SD might be interpreted as the most severe presentation of TOS and TIS.

5.5 Diagnostics

Diagnostic judgement on a therapy-resistant dystrophy depends on exact anamnesis, also focusing on predisposing causes, such as surgical procedures; injuries at work, in sports, traffic or accidents at home; inflammatory process; and cardiac disease. The development of the disease from the view of the patient, the duration of the symptoms and the kind of treatment received are important. It has to be found out whether the patient is sufficiently treated with pain medication or whether medication is only provided on demand, as this is essential for the prognosis of the disease. Invasive procedures as acupuncture, blockades of the brachial plexus and the stellate ganglion and i.v. regional blockades with guanethidine (Hannington-Kiff 1977) have to be inquired about as well.

5.5.1 Tabular Documentation of Pathologic Findings at the Upper Extremity

In order to compile a complete evaluation of all pathologic findings at the shoulder girdle, the region of the elbow and the forearm as well as the hand and to document the important preoperative findings essential for follow-up, the development of a tabular documentation is highly recommended (Fig. 5.7). It should include all pain localizations, neurological findings and other results of examination, such as articular function, comparing circumferences, examination of the volume of both hands (dip test) and the venous run-in pressure. Apart from colour of the skin and temperature and also strength and the extent of edema, different qualities of pain including allodynia and results of different tests and sympathetic block should be documented.

P.-No	Name First name	Date of Birth	Diagnosis	1. Examination
	Address:			
	Tel.			Reexamination
Anamnesis:				
			Op. right at:	Op. right at:

Lokal finding:*	preop.: r. l.	postop.: r. l.	R.Examinations				
			Hand - Thorax aperture – Cervical spine				
OCC. neuralgia							
SCS			Fu. Phlebo.: Subclavian vein				
ICS							
Triceps of arm			Angio.: Subclavian artery				
Brachial plexus							
Supraspinous fossa			**Longfingerfunction**				
Infraspinous fossa							
Accessory nerve			Deficit	D_2	D_3	D_4	D_5
Coracoid proc.			Flex. preop.				
Acromion			postop.				
Great tub. of humerus			Ext. preop.				
Deltoid. muscle insertion			postop.				
Hiaties ni. radialis			**Joint mobility**				
TE			Joints**	preop.: r. l.		postop.: r. l.	
Posterior pain area			SG/Abd.				
Rad. Tunnel syn.. of the Level of rad. head			EJ Flex.				
Supinatorcanal			Ext.				
Neuralgia of PIN			WJ Flex.				
R. superfic. ni. rad.			Ext.				
Styloiditis radii			r.	Circumference		l.	
N. cut. antebrach. posterior			preop.	postop.	cm	preop.	postop.
Styloiditis ulnae					OA		
Brachiorad muscle - ISTP					EL		
TV Wrist dorsalis					UA		
TV de Quervain					HW		
TV Carpalcanal					MH		

*Judging of pain (after VAS s. Tab. 11) and neurological findings: minimal = ((+)) slight (+).
strong = +, very strong = ++
**SJ = Shoulder joint, EJ = Elbow joint, WJ = Wrist joint, MH = Middle hand

Fig. 5.7 Examination sheet for patients with TOS and CRPS I

Lokal finding:*	preop.: r. l.	postop.: r. l.	Hand volume - Dipping test			
Median-CS			r		(ml)	l
GE			preop.	postop.	preop.	postop.
N. cut. antebrachii med.						
Sensib.: D1, 2, 3, 4, 5			Venous inlet pressure			
TV: D1, 2, 3, 4, 5			r		(cmH₂O)	l
Rough power						
Hand-FA-Ederma			Therapeutic blocks			
Scin color			Ggln. stellatum:			
Scin temperature			Brachial plexus:			
Resting pain			Guanethidin:			
Tender. to touch / Allodynia			Focus:		Pill:	
Tender. to pressure			Laboratory values:			
Pain of motion			Glucose:		Blood count:	
Hyperhidrosis			Lever values:			
Trophic disorders			ESR:		CRP:	
Test methods:	preop.: r. l.	postop.: r. l.	AST:		Rh.-Factor:	
Wear tests			Renal values:			
Abduction test by Roos			Urine:			
Elevation test			Sudeck Dystrophy (CRPS l)			
Redress. of Shoulder girdle			Age: Stage: Side:			
Accumulation test			Hospitalization by Doctor / Clinic:			
Ischemic test						
Sympathetic block						

Previous treatment and course.

Date: Medical examination by:

Fig. 5.7 (continued)

Table 5.2 CRPS I (1984–1991): shoulder girdle

Preoperative findings		Postoperative results			
$N_P = 10$ – follow-up – $N_{OP} = 10$	n	Excellent	Good	Fair	Unchanged
Occipital headache	4 →	2	–	1	1
Upper cervical syndrome	5 →	3	–	2	–
Lower cervical syndrome	8 →	5	1	1	1
Trapezius muscle	9 →	6	2	1	–
Brachial plexus	9 →	5	3	1	–
Supraspinous fossa	2 →	2	–	–	–
Infraspinous fossa	4 →	3	–	–	1
Accessory nerve	3 →	2	–	–	1
Coracoid process	6 →	3	–	2	1
Acromion	3 →	3	–	–	–
Greater tuberosity of humerus	6 →	4	2	–	–
Deltoid muscle insertion	4 →	3	1	–	–
Total	63 = 100 %	41 = 65.1 %	9 = 14.3 %	8 = 12.7 %	5 = 7.9 %

From Wilhelm (1997a, b)

Table 5.3 CRPS I (1984–1991): elbow and forearm

Preoperative findings		Postoperative results			
$N_P = 10$ – follow-up – $N_{OP} = 10$	n	Excellent	Good	Fair	Unchanged
Radial tunnel—proximal part	3 →	2	1	–	–
Radial tunnel—intermediate part	9 →	4	3	–	2
Radial tunnel—distal part	9 →	3	3	1	2
Lateral epicondylitis	10 →	4	3	1	2
Interosseous neuralgia	7 →	4	1	1	1
Radial styloiditis	7 →	5	2	–	–
Medial epicondylitis	1 →	1	–	–	–
Medial cutaneous nerve	3 →	2	1	–	–
Ulnar styloiditis	4 →	3	1	–	–
Brachioradialis muscle insertion	6 →	3	2	1	–
De Quervain disease	3 →	2	–	1	–
Total	62 = 100 %	33 = 53.2 %	17 = 27.4 %	5 = 8.1 %	7 = 11.3 %

From Wilhelm (1997a, b)

In acute dystrophy with strong pain, the test for damming and ischemia should only be performed exceptionally if essential for diagnostic reasons. For determination of stadium II and III of dystrophy, these examination methods are advisable.

The diagnosis of a neurogenous origin of Sudeck's dystrophy needs a diligent systematic examination of the upper extremity including the neck region. The most important examination results and the corresponding postoperative findings are presented in Tables 5.2, 5.3 and 5.4.

Mainly in peripheral nerve compression syndromes and out of reasons of differential diagnostics, there is an *indication for neurological examination*.

In order to confirm the diagnosis in any case after finishing the examinations, a *sympathetic block as stellate or plexus anaesthesia with naropine should be performed*, at

Table 5.4 CRPS I (1984–1991): hand

Preoperative findings	n	Postoperative results			
$N_P = 10$ – follow-up – $N_{OP} = 10$		Excellent	Good	Fair	Unchanged
Trophic and secretory disturbance	10 →	5	3	2	–
Hand edema	10 →	8	2	–	–
Increased	6 →	6	–	–	–
Skin temperature					
Decreased	4	1	2	1	–
Sensory disorders	10	6	4	–	–
Tactile pain	5 →	3	1	1	–
Palpation pain	10 →	8	1	1	–
Pain on movement	10 →	8	2	–	–
Rest pain	10 →	8	2	–	–
Decreased	5 →	2	1	2	–
Crude strength					
Not examined*	5 →	2	1	2	–
Median nerve compression	7 →	4	2	1	–
(No. 3, 4 and 7 not examined)	3 →	2	1	–	–
Soft tissue atrophy	1 →	–	1	–	–
Bone atrophy	9 →	5	3	1	–
Total	106 = 100 %	68 = 64.1 %	26 = 24.5 %	11 = 10.4 %	0

From Wilhelm (1997a, and b)
*Could not be tested because of pain.

the same time demonstrating the possible extent of a pain elimination by transaxillary decompression of the neurovascular bundle by additional sympathetic resection. X-rays of the hand in two levels and of the lower cervical spine in a.p. and half oblique are necessary as a standard. Here decalcifications of the hand bones and possible foramen stenoses can be seen. Special pictures of the upper thoracic aperture are important for surgery in order to see a cervical rib, an unusually long transverse process of the 7th cervical vertebra and a steep position or a hypoplasia of the 1st costa on time, as these structures might promote a compression of the brachial plexus and the subclavian artery.

A *cervical rib* or its fibrous and cartilaginous insertion at the first rib can even reduce the posterior scalenus gap leading to a shifting of the brachial plexus and the subclavian artery. A relieving high shoulder position already clinically hints at a cervical rib. Figure 5.8 gives a survey on varieties of cervical rib development.

Three-phase bone scintigraphy can be a helpful tool at the initial state I of the disease, but it is not specific! Other diseases as well can cause an accumulation in bone scan, like, for instance, inflammatory, infectious and tumour processes. But above all, this examination method cannot provide reliable information concerning prognosis, and it also cannot show whether the patient is suitable for a conservative or rather for a surgical therapy.

As the symptoms of Sudeck's dystrophy are strikingly similar to those of TOS, a functional phlebography, as obligatory in this syndrome, was also introduced as a

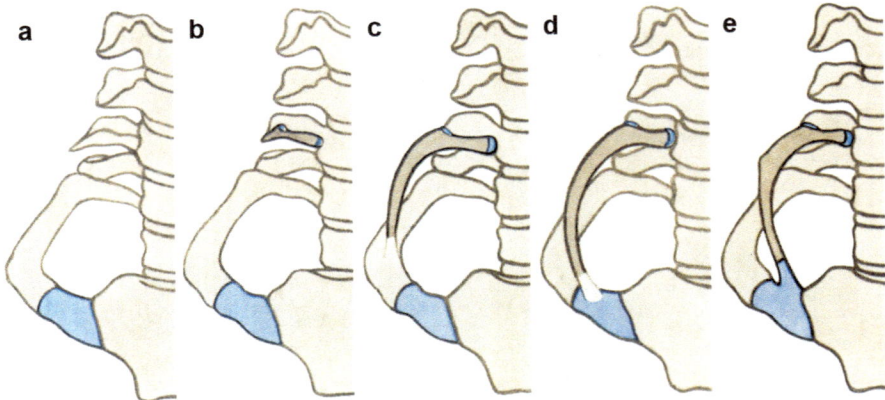

Fig. 5.8 (**a**) Varieties of cervical ribs, unusually long transverse process of the 7th cervical verte-bra. (**b**) The front section of the costotransverse process forms a rib brace, connected to the trans-verse process and the vertebra. (**c**) The rudimentary cervical costa exceeds the transverse process ending free; only in 5 % there is a connection to the first costa. (**d**) The cervical costa reaches the 1st costa in fibrous, cartilaginous or osseous manner. (**e**) The cervical costa behaves like a thoracic costa. It reaches the sternal manubrium by its cartilage melted with the 1st costa. (From von Lanz and Wachsmuth 1955)

diagnostic tool in Sudeck's dystrophy to check the conditions of run-in at the sub-clavian vein in this disease as well, hoping to find a logical explanation for the acute edema in this dystrophy.

In this disease functional phlebography is performed considering the pain limit in adduction and abduction of the arm, if possible in 0–60–0° in lying or sitting position. Pictures in elevation are not essential in Sudeck and should be avoided due to the strong pain connected.

Ultravist 300 is used as contrast medium in a bolus of 30 ml/contrast series.

- *Injection follows after the application of a tourniquet into the basilica vein in order to not endanger the judgement of reflux into the cephalic vein in an essential disturbance at the subclavian vein.*

In 25 out of 26 patients with resistant dystrophy surgically treated by the author, a striking impairment of the venous run-in at the subclavian vein with reflux into the cephalic vein and in massive changes also in combination with a collateral circle was seen in phlebography.

The venous stasis can be determined numerically by measuring the venous run-in pressure in the sitting patient (Dunant 1987). First the pressure in the axillary vein compared to the level of the atria is determined using an infusion machine for saline solution. After pushing forward the catheter pressure conditions at the subclavian stenosis and finally of the brachiocephalic vein are determined. Here prestenotic pressures up to 35 cm H_2O can be found if a collateral circle is missing, whereas pressure can fall down to 0 cm H_2O in the stenotic area. Pressures in the upper vena cava in a healthy patient are up to -3 cm H_2O and below. In a massive collateral circle, even a lower pressure of run-in can be found (Fig. 5.9). There also is a slighter hand edema in these cases.

Fig. 5.9 X-ray of i.v. pressure measurement at axillary vein, subclavian vein and right brachiocephalic vein. Due to good collateral blood supply, there is normal pressure in axillary vein

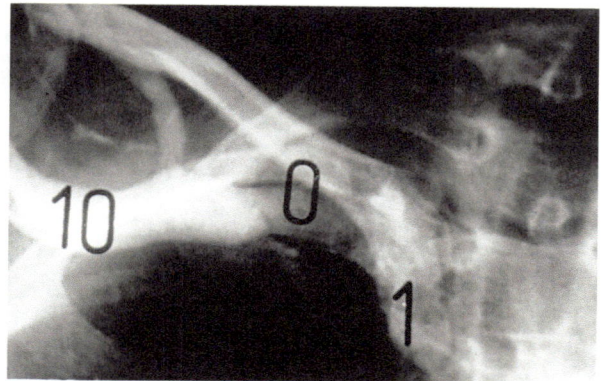

Fig. 5.10 Preoperative phlebography of left subclavian vein (*asterisk*). Broad a.p. compression by endothoracic fascia. Significant compression of axillary vein by strong minor pectoral muscle (*3 arrows*), preventing the development of a reflux into the cephalic vein and the development of a collateral circulation by decrease of pressure in the axillary and subclavian vein (*** and *VS*)

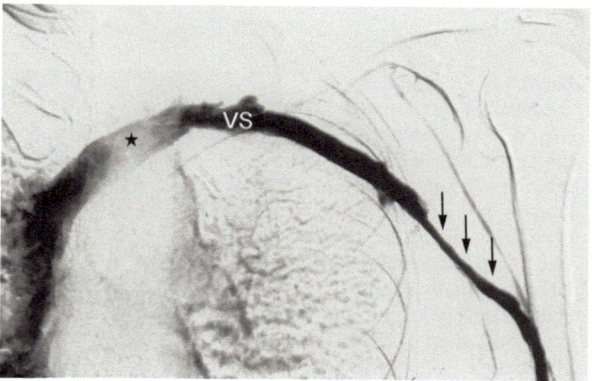

Determination of the venous run-in pressure can also check the postoperative result of a successful decompression of the subclavian vein if postoperative phlebography should be difficult to interpret. This is also true for the postoperative determination of hand volume and circumference.

5.5.2 Phlebography of Subclavian Vein

Phlebographic findings in Sudeck's dystrophy can be divided into six basic presentations, being:

1. *Posterior-anterior compression of the subclavian vein* caused by pressure of a strongly developed endothoracic fascia (Sibson fascia) with and without reflux into the cephalic vein and development of a collateral circle (Figs. 5.10 and 5.11).

2. *Stripe-formed vertical compression* caused by thoracic artery and phrenic nerve enclosed in the Sibson fascia. Figure 5.12 shows this compression combined with a trough-shaped impression in the inferior part of the vessel, caused by the

Fig. 5.11 Preoperative presentation of a broad a.p. stenosis caused by the endothoracic fascia on the right (*white arrow*) with reflux into the cephalic vein (*small arrow*) and collateral circle (*large black arrow*). (From Wilhelm 1997a, b, with kind permission from Thieme)

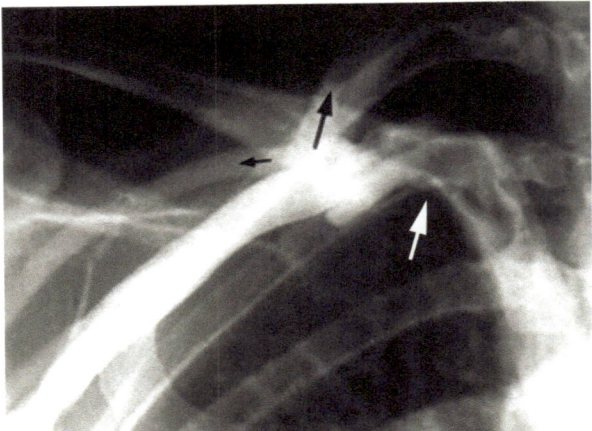

Fig. 5.12 Preoperative presentation of a stripe-shaped, vertical stenosis of the right subclavian vein (*VS*) caused by the internal thoracic artery and phrenic nerve structures in the Sibson fascia (*asterisk*). Additional inferior compression by anterior scalene muscle and tendinous origin of subclavian muscle (*white arrow*). Significant reflux into a double cephalic vein (*VC, two black arrows*). (From Wilhelm 1997b, with kind permission from Thieme)

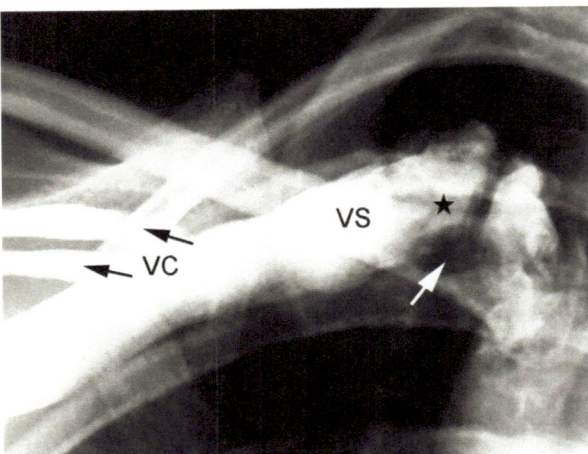

tendinous origin of the subclavian muscle (white arrow). There is a strong reflux into a duplicate cephalic vein (Fig. 5.12).

Further lateral of this compression, other phlebographies show partial stripe-shaped and also vertically ordered compressions caused by a prominent ligamentary front rim of the anterior scalene muscle.

3. *Filiform stenosis of the subclavian vein*: In Fig. 5.14 a stenosis with reflux into the cephalic vein is shown in Sudeck's dystrophy, state II. Figure 5.15 shows the postoperative run-in into the left subclavian vein. No reflux can be seen any more.

4. *Stenosis of the subclavian vein in cone shape*: In Fig. 5.16 phlebography shows this stenosis in a dystrophy for 13 years, caused only by a very strong Sibson fascia (intraoperative finding). The technique presented here can also determine the extent of stenosis, 70.9 % in this case. (This picture was kindly provided by Prof. Eisenschenk, Berlin-Marzahn.)

Fig. 5.13 Shows free venous run-in after transaxillary decompression of the subclavian vein. The former localisation of the stenosis (*white arrow*) is no more recognizable (postoperative result after vanishing of edema Figs. 5.36 and 5.37; functional result Table 5.9, patient 7)

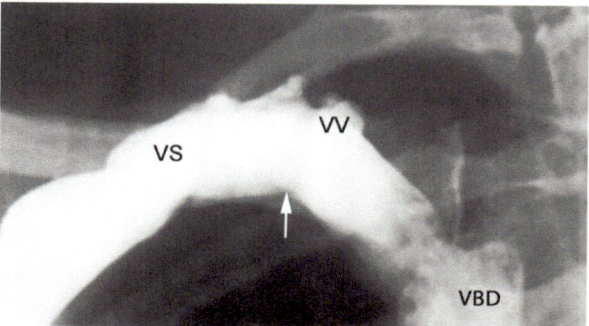

Fig. 5.14 Phlebographic proof of a filiform stenosis of the subclavian vein (*VS*) with reflux into cephalic vein (*VC*) in adduction of arm, *VA* axillary vein. (From Wilhelm 2007). Localisation of subclavian vein (*VS*) see Fig. 5.15, *black arrow*

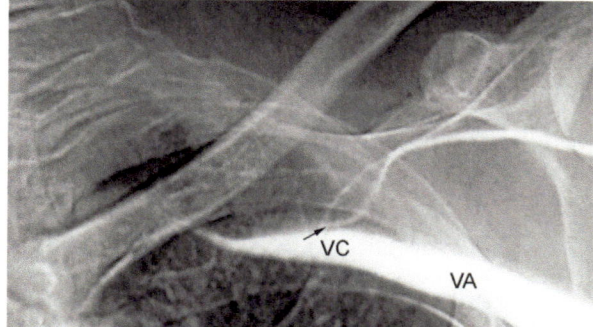

Fig. 5.15 Postoperatively the stenosis seen in Fig. 5.14 is not seen any more (*white arrow, VS*), as well as the reflux into the cephalic vein. *VA* axillary vein, *BVVS* valvular bulbus of subclavian vein (From Wilhelm 2007)

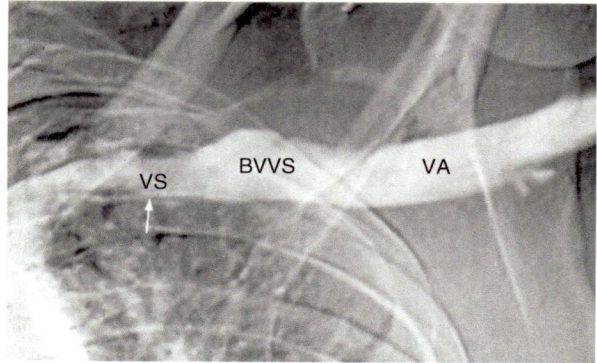

5. *Circular stenosis of the subclavian vein*: Caused by the subclavian muscle in the upper area of the vessel, by the anterior scalene muscle at the lower side and by the endothoracic fascia in p.–a. direction (Fig. 5.17).
6. *Non-thrombotic obstruction of the subclavian vein*: Figure 5.18 shows a finding with collateral circle and reflux into the cephalic vein. In this case compression of the vessel is caused by the anterior scalene muscle and the subclavian muscle as well as by a strong endothoracic fascia. The patient did not agree on a postoperative control.

Fig. 5.16 Conical stenosis of subclavian vein caused by strong Sibson fascia. *BVVS* valvular bulbus of subclavian vein. (From Wilhelm 2007)

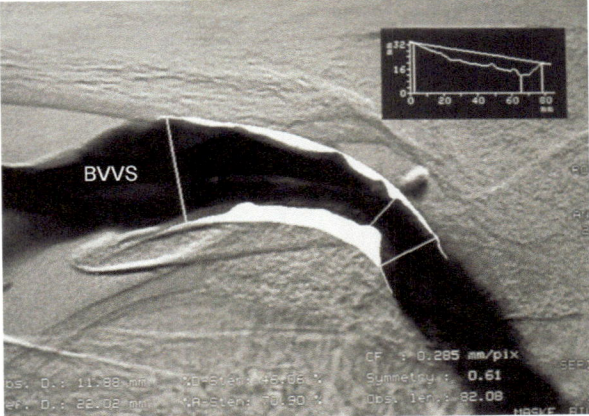

Fig. 5.17 Preoperative phlebographic finding of a subclavian vein circular stenosis (*white arrow*) with collateral circulation (*thick arrows*: × 2 long, × 1 short) and reflux into cephalic vein (*VC*, *thin black arrow*); picture in abduction of the arm. (From Wilhelm 1997b, with kind permission from Thieme)

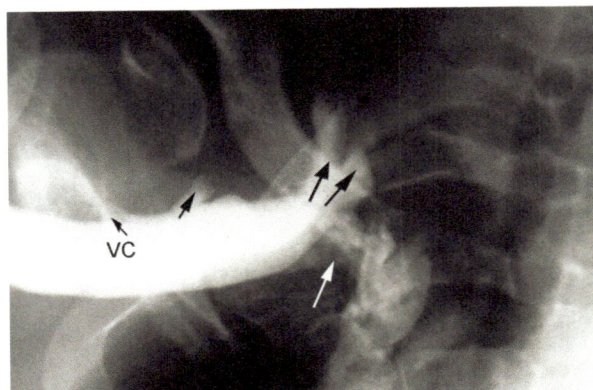

Fig. 5.18 Non-thrombotic obstruction of subclavian vein (*VS*) with pronounced collateral circulation (*bow-shaped arrow*) and reflux into cephalic vein (*straight arrow*). Intraoperative findings and remarks *cf.* text. (From Wilhelm 1997b, with kind permission from Thieme)

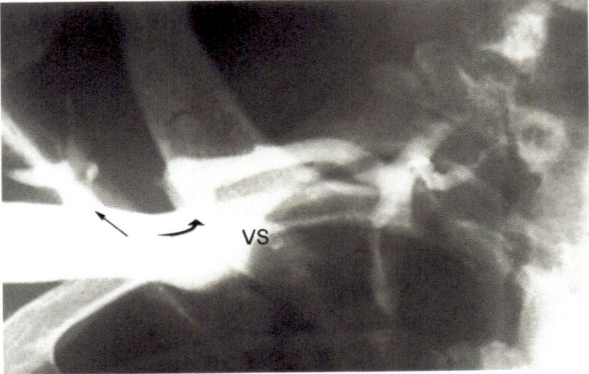

The good postoperative course shows decompression resulted in an excellent venous run-in. After finishing postoperative treatment, the patient was able to return to his former profession as a locksmith in completely free articular function and with restitution of crude strength (postoperative function Figs. 5.9, 5.38, 5.39 and 5.40, patient 4).

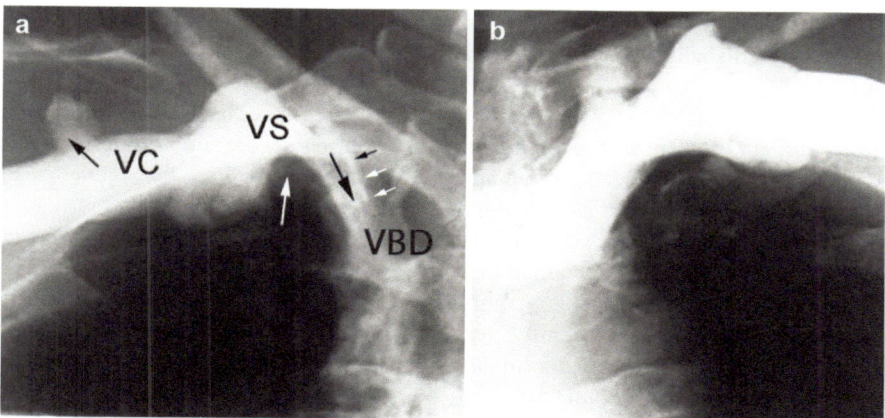

Fig. 5.19 (**a**) Phlebographic finding in Sudeck's Dystrophy with inferior compression of subclavian vein (*VS*) and reflux into cephalic vein (*VC, left arrow*). Influx into right brachio-cephalic vein
(*VBD, thick arrow*) also stenotically changed, limited by 3 *small arrows*. Cause might mainly be a
compression via sibson's fascia. (**b**) Normal phlebography of subclavian vein on the healthy side.
(From Wilhelm 2007)

In Fig. 5.19 findings in Sudeck's dystrophy on the right side and on the healthy
left side are presented. Rarely there is a pathologic change of the subclavian vein on
both sides with dystrophy. Since 1982, this was seen in 2 patients.

Development of collateral circles is accomplished by little branches of the subclavian
vein, by the acromial venous rete and especially by the transverse neck veins and the
superficial cervical comitant veins, leading into the external jugular vein next to the subclavian vein. Also connections of the superficial cervical comitant veins with the
profound cervical vein serve for venous run-off, as well as the intercostal venous system
via internal thoracic comitant veins. By reduction of pressure at the subclavian vein and
by reflux into the cephalic vein, these paths of venous run-in are only rarely seen in
phlebography. Clinically the collateral circle can be seen macroscopically in an increase
of presentation of subcutaneous vessels of the upper thoracic region. Pectoral veins and
perforating branches of the internal thoracic vein also contribute to this circle.

The run-in of the congested venous blood is easier at the neck as the veins of the
neck in the transition area to the thorax are held open by braces and also experience
the suck effect of the mediastinal negative pressure. The veins of the neck are no
pressure veins, but sucking veins (von Lanz and Wachsmuth 1959).

The small veins of the neck are only comitant veins, attached to their corresponding arterial vessels, thus supported by pulse pressure. Consequently the transverse
neck comitant veins have the same course as the transverse neck artery, then leading
as one vessel stem into the subclavian vein lateral of the frontal scalene gap.

In CRPS I patients the stenosis of the subclavian vein usually can already be seen
in adduction, whereas in healthy people this mainly is the case in arm elevation.
This does not mean, however, that "healthy persons" suffer from venous stenosis.
This finding is seen mainly in trophically disturbed hands with impairment of fist
closure in the morning, in not so rare relapse after a correct median decompression
and in patients who complain about hand swelling and increased venous filling at

the back of the hand after garden work or after a surgical procedure. Here the cause as well is a disbalance between a high arterial run-in and simultaneous impairment of venous run-in by a subclavian vein stenosis.

Figures 5.5 and 5.6 show an example, being a hereditary "hand-finger syndrome" after surgery of a Dupuytren contracture. In this case a severe subclavian stenosis of 75 % was found as the cause of edema.

- In hand edema always keep in mind a venous stenosis.

In this context it has to be mentioned again that a stenosis of the subclavian vein was found and also examined histologically as the cause of idiopathic median nerve compression (Fig. 5.1). Median compression by edema also develops after injuries of any kind at the upper extremity, during pregnancy, during continuous medication with oral contraceptives, endocrinous diseases (acromegaly and solid edema) and after creation of an AV fistula.

5.5.3 Arteriography of Subclavian Artery

Apart from typical findings in clinical examination especially the proof of the irritation responsible at the lower plexus roots, at the intervertebral foramina and the "thoracic outlet", radiologically seen in cervical spine x-rays and in angiography of the subclavian artery point towards an elevated sympathetic activity in CRPS I.

An indication for arteriography is given only in stenotic noise, pulse weakening, and blood pressure differences of 20 mmHg and more, as well as in suspicion of an aneurysm, in obstruction of the peripheral vessels and in Raynaud's disease. There are rare events when this exam is also performed in dystrophy for diagnostic and scientific reasons, as this method in the meantime has been replaced by the much less invasive intravenous subtraction angiography (DSA), in special cases also being performed as intra-arterial technique.

Arteriographic examinations were done in 7 out of 26 patients. Pathologic findings at the subclavian artery were as follows:

1. Dislocation of the subclavian artery in cranial and posterior direction: Figure 5.20 shows an example. In a neck rib there is a transposition of the artery as well as of the brachial plexus to the upper front (intraoperative findings).
2. Narrow band-shaped compression of the subclavian artery: In these cases compression is caused either by a ligamentary changed anterior scalene muscle (intraoperative finding) or by a fibrous rudiment of the minimus scalene muscle (Fig. 5.21).
3. Circumscribed inferior compression of the subclavian artery: The main cause of the impression depicted in Fig. 5.22 is a hypertrophic anterior scalene muscle. Similar changes can also be caused by a strong subclavian muscle.
4. Lengthy stenosis of the subclavian artery: The stenosis pictured in Fig. 5.23 was caused by compressive effect of the anterior scalene muscle (white arrows) and a minimus scalene muscle (black arrows)—intraoperative finding.

The arteriographic findings demonstrated, together with the impairment of the subclavian artery found intraoperatively, show that not only the lower plexus roots, as already known, but also the artery mentioned have to be regarded as a starting point of sympathetic efferences. The impairment of this artery by fibromuscular

Fig. 5.20 Arteriographic finding of right subclavian artery with vessel dislocation in cranial and posterior direction (*small arrows*), caused by anterior scalene muscle. *AA* axillar artery; *AS* subclavian artery; *TTC* thyrocervical trunk; *AV* vertebral artery; *ACC* common carotid artery; *ATI* internal thoracic artery; *TBC* brachiocephalic trunk

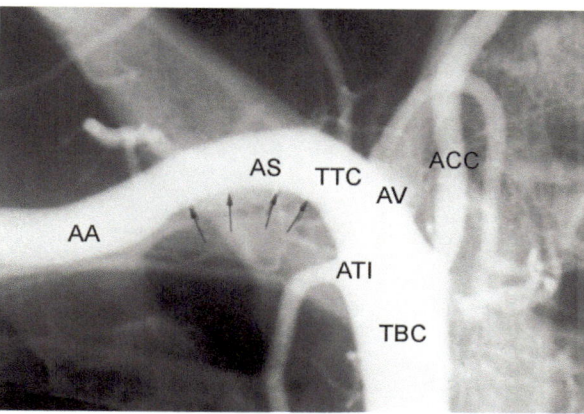

Fig. 5.21 Band-shaped stenosis of subclavian artery (*AS, white arrow*) caused by anterior scalene muscle; explanation of headings in Fig. 5.20

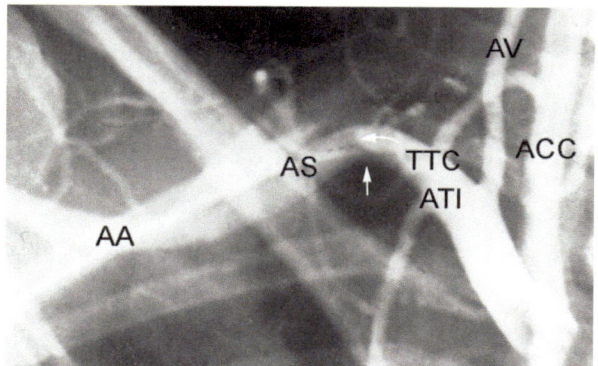

Fig. 5.22 Inferior compression of subclavian artery (*AS*), caused by hypertrophic anterior scalene muscle with additional impairment of the vessel by a minimus scalene muscle (*white arrow*); explanation of headings in Fig. 5.20

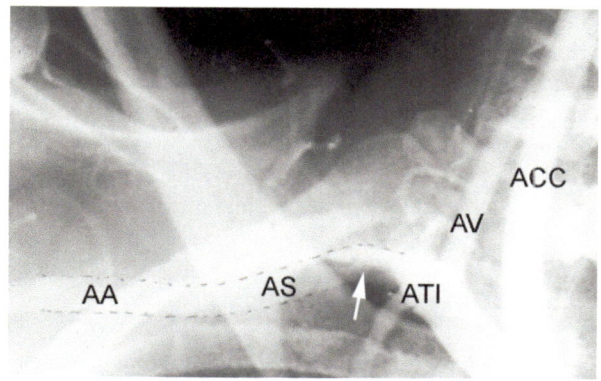

structures as seen in Table 5.5 automatically leads to an ongoing irritation of the postganglion sympathetic fibres running along the subclavian artery and the axillary artery. These can be followed macroscopically until the anterior section of the shoulder joint and the subcoracoid region, explaining pain projection into this region in CRPS I as well as in *TOS, falsely known as the so-called coracoiditis.*

Fig. 5.23 Lengthy stenosis of subclavian artery by compressive anterior scalene muscle effect (*white arrows*) and a minimus scalene muscle (*black arrows*); explanation of headings in Fig. 5.20

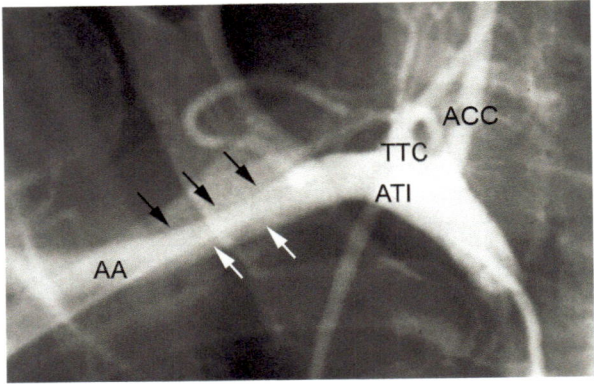

Table 5.5 M. Sudeck (1984–1991 and 2000–2002) - Intra operative findings (Nop. = 20) irritating and compressing structures

V. subclavia		A. subclavia		Lower plexus roots	
M. scalenus anterior	12	M. scalenus anterior	15	Costa I	7
M. subclavius	4	M. scalenus minimus	4	Fibrous structures	4
Lig. costoclaviculare	4	Lig. pleurovertebrale	10	M. scalenus minimus	5
Fascia endothoracica Lig. pleurovertebrale	15 3	Arcades and fibrous replacement of M.scal. minimus	9	Cervical rib	0[a]
Stenosis of V. subclavia	20	Poststen. aneurysm	0	Substantial Damage	7
		Dislocation of A. subclavia	7		

[a]In the above mentioned periods a cervical rib could only be found in a conservatively treated patient.

5.5.4   Brachial Plexus and Intraoperative Findings

Irritations and compressions of the brachial plexus are mostly caused by the sharp inner rim of costa 1 and by basal fibrous arcade-shaped structures, which may also run below the subclavian artery. In 7 out of 20 patients, there was a substantial damage of the lower plexus roots in the shape of subepineural haematoma and groove-shaped impressions. Frequently there are also irritations by fibrous structures and a strong minimus scalene muscle.

Table 5.5 shows a survey concerning irritating and compressing structures at the subclavian vessels and the brachial plexus.

5.5.5   Differential Diagnosis

In differential diagnosis CRPS I differs from causalgia (CRPS II), the pain localization of which is limited to the innervation area of the peripheral nerves affected, in contrast to Sudeck's dystrophy. Superficial spontaneous pain and so-called allodynia without essential orthostatic reaction are characteristic. They cannot be influenced by the so-called ischaemia test. It is striking that optic, acoustic, emotional and especially sexual triggers can lead to intolerable increase of pain. Also causalgia is characterised by the lack of peripheral edema and changes in skin temperature. Distribution of pain can also concern the contralateral extremity, called alloparalgia.

- *In Sudeck's dystrophy similar findings are seen at the contralateral upper extremity and the leg of the same side. In the latter case the complaints disappear immediately after upper thoracic sympathetic resection.*

In differential diagnosis arthritic and especially posttraumatic and postoperative edema (Figs. 5.5 and 5.6) and thrombosis of the subclavian vein (Paget-von Schroetter syndrome) have to be seen. In case of doubt, also self-mutilation should be kept in mind. A non-removable cast of the fist and forearm can solve the problem.

5.6   Classification

The former classification of CRPS I in 3 states of disease was never proven statistically (Winkel and Blonder 2011) and was also not reliable in practical work. Since the introduction of subclavian vein phlebography, acute dystrophy can be divided into a conservatively treatable form with good prognosis and into a therapy-resistant form, depending on the phlebographic result. Here subclavian vein stenosis can be divided into a mild (0–<30 %), severe (30–<70 %) and most severe (70–100 %) form. Mild dystrophies are treated conservatively; the remaining two other forms should be treated conservatively only for 4–8 weeks; in the lack of success they should be treated surgically in the 2nd–3rd month.

Dystrophies treated conservatively (approximately 85–90 %; cf. Sect. 5.5.2) and those having to be treated surgically (cf. Sect.5.7).

Dystrophies treated conservatively for too long can experience destruction of the interneuroma cell core resulting in a loss of pain inhibitory function (cf. Sect. 5.11).

5.7   Indications and Contraindications

Indication for transaxillary decompression of the neurovascular bundle with upper thoracic extrapleural resection of the sympathetic tract including the first three ganglia is only given in therapy-resistant dystrophy and in extreme stenosis of the subclavian vein. It should be given earlier than 9 months after first diagnosed. In *subclavian vein stenosis of 50% and more*, surgery should be performed within 2–3 months in order to reach an excellent or good result, also to save the patient from longer postoperative treatment and pain, also taking care of his workplace. According to Roos (1977), transaxillary surgery in TOS can also be performed bilaterally at the same time with advantages for the patient.

The main *contraindication* is causalgia (CRPS II) as in this case the painful process is not caused by the thoracic outlet but by circumscribed injury of a peripheral nerve. Further on general contraindications for surgical procedures of similar extent are applicable.

Table 5.6 CRPS I (1984–1991 and 2000–2002): Surgical treatment in resistant cases ($n=20$)

Sex	$16 \times F: 4 \times M$
Age (21–73 years)	$\varnothing = 45$ years
Surgical procedures:	
TOS operation (technique of Roos)	Right: $15 \times$ left: $5 \times$
Op. with sympathectomy (upper thoracic resection[a] or neurotomy of communicating branches)	$15 \times$ (pat. 1; 3–10; 15, 16–20)
Op. with neurotomy of postganglionic branches	$4 \times$ (pat. 11–14)
Op. without sympathectomy	$1 \times$ (pat. 2)

From Wilhelm (2007)
Stage II: $16 \times$, Stage III: $4 \times$ (Pat. 5, 12, 13 and 15)
[a]OP with additional periarterial sympathectomy: $2 \times$

Whether and in how far the quite rare bilateral disease and patients presenting too late have a contraindication can only be decided in each single case. The memantine (AXURA) test (Sinis et al. 2006) mentioned can help with this decision.

Memantine is used in small doses and gradually increased:

- 1st week: ½ tab. (5 mg) in the morning
- 2nd week: $2 \times$½ tab. (10 mg) 5–0–5 mg
- 3rd week (15 mg) 10–0–5 mg
- 4th week (20 mg) 10–0–10 mg
- From the 5th week on, the dose can be increased to 25 mg if tolerated well 15–0–10 mg.
- From the 6th week on, the maximum dose is 30 mg 15–0–15 mg.

As soon as the patient reports an improvement of pain, dose can be reduced consecutively, also in patients with side effects. In the first case there is an indication for surgery; in the second case there is only very limited indication (Table 5.6).

5.8   Surgical Treatment of Resistant Cases

5.8.1 History

Multiple fasciotomies as published by Ehlert (1974) *are a milestone in surgical treatment of Sudeck's dystrophy*, which are based on the supposition of a subfascial increase of pressure. This procedure does not only lead to immediate removal of pain, but it also prevents from results of this dystrophy. The identical effect was also accomplished by Sudmann and Sundsfjord in 1984 by an extensive fasciotomy of the forearm flexion side with simultaneous median decompression.

As symptoms of CRPS I are strikingly similar to those of a thoracic outlet syndrome, phlebographies were performed in these dystrophies as well, showing an impairment of venous run-in caused by stenosis at the subclavian vein. This finding led to the decision to also surgically treat therapy-resistant dystrophy. The first three successfully surgically treated dystrophies were already reported in 1985 (Wilhelm and Wilhelm).

5.8.2   Informed Patient Consent

Prior to conservative or surgical treatment, the help-seeking, scared and often misunderstood patient needs to be informed about the real cause of this organic disease. With regard to the patient, additional discussion of a possible significance of changes in the central nervous system should be omitted on purpose, as there is great danger that the patient has the conception that changes in psychic regard might be seen as a possible cause of the disease by physicians and hand therapists! The question whether central changes are a triggering cause or only a secondary phenomenon has not been answered yet.

Family members should join in the health education before the informed consent in order to be instructed about the nature of the disease, the methods of treatment and which course can be expected. Only then the patient will receive the understanding necessary for his situation in his family and a feeling of well-being and care.

In some cases it also makes sense to inform the employer after consent of the family. This is also true for those health insurances not allowing for costs of a hospital stay or expensive pain medication.

Explanation of the surgical principle and both differing methods of sympathetic eliminations in the upper thoracic area (resection of ganglia T I–III or neurotomy of communicating branches).

Resection of intercostobrachial nerve for prophylactic elimination of pain at the upper arm is mainly implicated in severe old dystrophy with significant painful stiffness of mobility in the shoulder joint.

5.8.2.1 Possible Remaining Results
1. Blepharophimosis (Horner syndrome), mostly transient, improvement even possible after many years
2. Dryness of skin at the arm, chest, neck and face area on the side surgically treated
3. Decrease of sensibility at the inner and extension side of the upper arm as a result of cutting the intercostobrachial nerve

5.8.2.2 Complications
1. Intraoperative bleeding: Bleeding from the 1st intercostal artery.
2. Infection, embolism despite precautions.
3. Injury of forearm nerve bundle (hand weakness!).
4. Rupture of costal pleura over cupula pleurae. Smaller lesions are harmless, not needing a suture. Larger lesions are sutured.
5. Lesion of cupula pleurae with loss of air: Intraoperative suture. Postoperative pneumothorax: treatment by thoracic suction drainage.
6. Secondary compression of the arm vein possible by excessive scarring.

7. Postoperative development of effusion in the pleural space. In the lesion of the costal pleura drainage of the effusion via intrapleural drainage (lower head position), otherwise treatment by puncture or drainage.
8. Conjunctivitis (sandy sensation).
9. Stress on costal pleura by effusion possible.
10. Postoperative development of *intercostal neuralgia with pain in the upper thoracic area, worsening in inspiration*. Conservative treatment, *if persisting, surgical treatment by neurotomy* to relax the intercostal nerves.

5.8.2.3 No Guarantee for Success

A guarantee for success in pain improvement and joint motion in the operated arm cannot be given. However, there is a good chance in up to 90 % if the procedure is performed during the first 3–9 months after the start of conservative treatment. In advanced therapy-resistant disease with painful stiffness of the shoulder joint, surgery can only be recommended with precaution.

Even after an immediate good postoperative result, lack of relaxation and unexpected traction damage of the brachial plexus can even result in an extreme deterioration of postoperative findings and pain measurement. Further disturbance of the pain-inhibiting system of the dorsal horn of spinal cord synapses is primarily responsible, depending on duration and extension of the painful process even leading to an absolute therapy resistance.

In order to preserve the success, the operated arm needs to be placed in abduction (functional position) during the night and on an abduction pillow with tension band effect during daytime, mainly preventing traction damage of the arm nerve plexus. Consequently carrying bags, shaking hands and friendly clapping on the shoulder absolutely have to be prevented. This also applies to shaking while driving a car and using public transportation.

Training of joint motion in the operated arm may only be undertaken actively under medical and physiotherapeutic surveillance, aiming at therapy being accomplished by the patient himself.

Informed consent to surgery should not only be signed according to usual guidelines but also by a witness, if possible.

5.8.3   Instruments

- Lamp, magnifying glasses, if needed
- Knife for single use
- Fine electric knife
- 1 Preparation scissors 28 cm; BC 281; Aeskulap
- 1 Preparation scissors 23 cm; 11- 943–23; Martin
- 1 Needle holder 23 cm; BM o36R; Aeskulap
- 2 Overholt 28/27 cm; Nr. 4; Ullrich

- 1 Corn tongs 20 cm; BF U47; Aeskulap
- 1 Wire cutter 20 cm; FO 640; Aeskulap
- 1 Curved Luer bone rongeur 28 cm according to Wilhelm; Ullrich Co., Ulm
- 1 Rib raspatory long angled 30 cm according to ROOS; Ullrich Co.
- 1 Rib raspatory short angled 20 cm
- 2 Rib raspatory round (right/left) 17 cm each
- 1 Raspatory round 18.5 cm; FK 350 Aeskulap
- 1 TOS spatula according to Roos 35 cm; Ullrich Co.
- 1 "Grandfather" liver-spatula; BT 758 Aeskulap
- 1 Surgical tweezers 30 cm; BD 563 Aeskulap
- 2 Surgical Ewald tweezers fine, medium; Fehling Co./Aeskulap
- 2 Anatomic Ewald tweezers fine, medium; Fehling Co./Aeskulap
- 1 Anatomic tweezers 30 cm; 12- 100–30; Martin
- 1 Anatomic tweezers 30 cm; 24- 388–30; Martin
- 2 Langenbeck retractors 14 cm (length of spatula); BT 528; Aeskulap
- 2 Langenbeck retractors 10 cm (length of spatula); EAZ-5; Fehling

5.8.4 Surgical Technique of Transaxillary Decompression of Neurovascular Bundle and Extrapleural Resection of Upper Sympathetic Trunk, Respectively, Neurotomy of Communicating Branches Running Towards the Lower Plexus Roots

The transaxillary access is the technically most simple and also the most tolerable procedure for the patient (Schink 1972, Roos 1977).

Side position of patient (Fig. 5.24). After preparation and covering the surgical site, the arm wrapped in sterile cloth is held in abduction by the second assistant and is elevated cautiously, moved to the back or to the front, if needed. Longer extension absolutely has to be prevented due to danger of plexus damage. Diagonal skin incision at the third costa extends from the front rim of the dorsal latissimus muscle to the lower rim of the major pectoral muscle, directly below the border of axillary hair. After incision of the superficial fascia, the thoracoepigastric vessel and lymphatic system are prepared, isolated and cut after ligation. Afterwards further preparation follows along the lateral thoracic wall, saving the thoracodorsal nerve and its vessels leading to the frontal inner side of the dorsal latissimus muscle, as well as the long thoracic nerve running over the anterior serratus muscle.

In *CRPS I* in contrast to thoracic outlet syndrome, the intercostobrachial nerve should be cut to spare the patient from ongoing and sometimes intolerable dysaesthesia of the inner and dorsal side of the upper arm, especially since the loss of sensibility after surgery has never been complained about after adequate preoperative explanation; on the contrary the limitation of sensibility is rather regarded as harmless.

Fig. 5.24 Positioning of patient on the side, arm held by second assistant, type of incision. (From Wilhelm and Wilhelm 1985, with kind permission from Thieme)

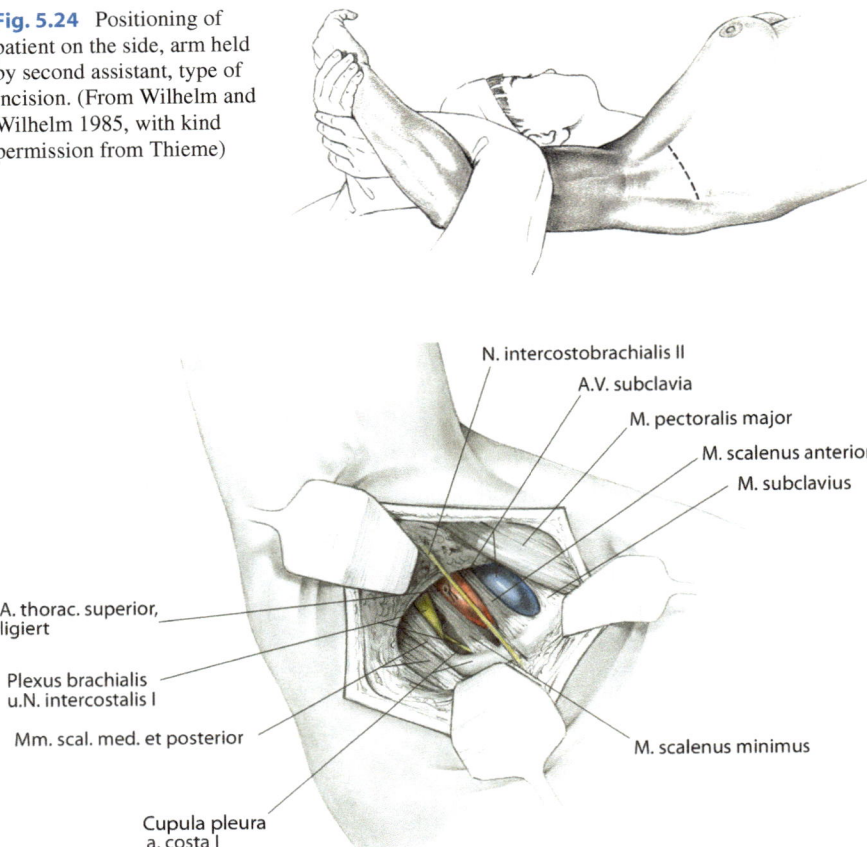

N. intercostobrachialis II

A.V. subclavia

M. pectoralis major

M. scalenus anterior

M. subclavius

A. thorac. superior, ligiert

Plexus brachialis u.N. intercostalis I

Mm. scal. med. et posterior

M. scalenus minimus

Cupula pleura a. costa I

Fig. 5.25 Presentation of 1st costa and anterior and posterior scalenus gap. (From Wilhelm and Wilhelm 1985, with kind permission from Thieme)

After further preparation in cranial direction, you see variations of the supreme thoracic vessels, springing from the axillary vessels and running into the muscles of the 1st intercostal space. These vessels have to be ligated twice and then cut, with an additional anchor for the distal vessel stump by a situated suture into the muscle.

Now the way to the 1st costa is clear, it is prepared from the tendinous origin of the subclavian muscle up to the level of the medius scalene muscle insertion (Figs. 5.25 and 5.28).

The tendinous origin of the subclavian muscle at the 1st costa insertion of cartilage, gripping the frontal basal area of the subclavian vein, while the insertion of the anterior scalene muscle runs below this vessel from the scalene tuberculum, receives special attention. The subclavian vein then runs below the clavicula and the subclavius muscle in front of the anterior scalene muscle over the 1st costa connected to the periosteum of the 1st rib and the tendinous fascial quiver of the subclavius

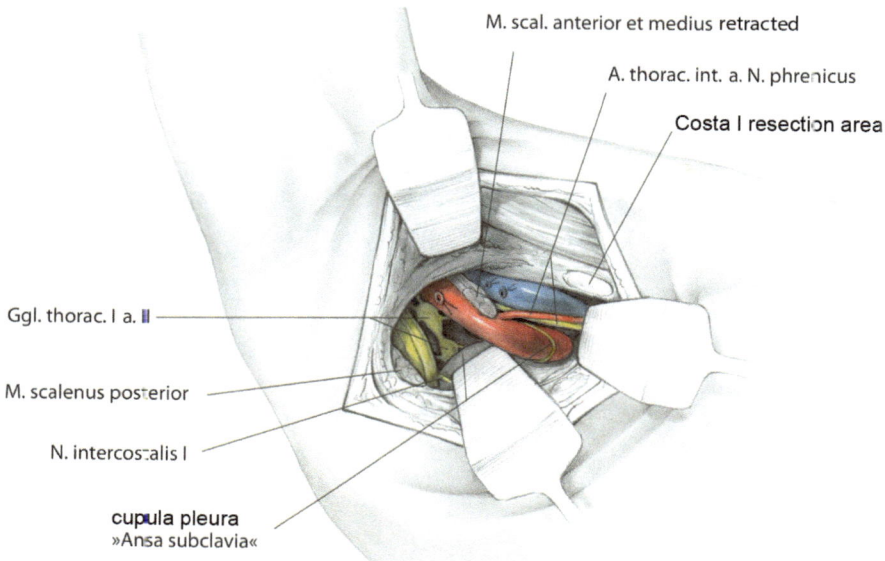

M. scal. anterior et medius retracted

A. thorac. int. a. N. phrenicus

Costa I resection area

Ggl. thorac. I a. II

M. scalenus posterior

N. intercostalis I

cupula pleura
»Ansa subclavia«

Fig. 5.26 Status post resection of 1st costa and desinsertion of anterior and medius scalene muscles (retracted) and resection of scalenus minimus muscle. (From Wilhelm and Wilhelm 1985, with kind permission from Thieme)

muscle, permanently keeping the venous lumen open to favour venous flow back. Still the subclavian vein can nevertheless be impressed in hypertrophic and tendinous changes of the anterior scalene muscle and its anterior portion of origin at the posterior and inferior side on its way. This also applies to the subclavius muscle, being the main cause of superior impression of the subclavian vein. Also accessory fibromuscular structures from the anterior scalene muscle and its medial side have to be kept in mind in this area.

The dorsal axillary gap may present an additional minimus scalene muscle dividing the subclavian artery and the brachial plexus, possibly irritating both structures, especially in hypertrophy and sharply edged border as well as in development of a fibrous rudiment.

Then the anterior scalene muscle is sharply cut 1 cm proximal to its insertion over an overholt forceps (Figs. 5.26, 5.27 and 5.28), loosening the subclavian vein from its fascial quiver. The fibrous arcade-shaped structures at the inner side of the first costa have to be taken care of, the course below the subclavian artery and the brachial plexus, and can also irritate (Table 5.5).

The tendinous subclavian origin is then cut in diagonal direction and completely resected in case of a significant superior impression of the subclavian vein. Then resection of a possibly existent minimus scalene muscle and loosening of the medius scalene muscle diligently preserving the brachial plexus follow. This muscle is directly cut from the 1st costa in order to present a good soft tissue underfeeding of the lower plexus roots at the end of surgery (Figs. 5.25 and 5.29). In separating the

Fig. 5.27 Presentation of a strong ligamentary change of an anterior scalene muscle, MSA subclavian vein below right retractor. (From Wilhelm and Wilhelm 1985, with kind permission from Thieme)

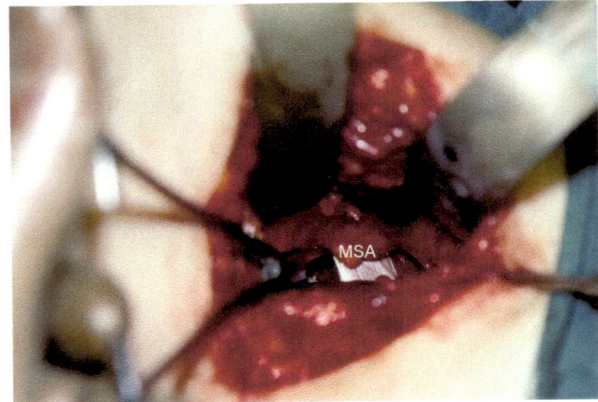

Fig. 5.28 Intraoperative presentation of anatomic structures at the anterior and posterior scalene gap. *V* subclavian vein, *A* subclavian artery, *P* brachial plexus; *asterisk*: insertion of anterior scalene muscle at 1st rib and 2 *asterisks* medial scalene muscle

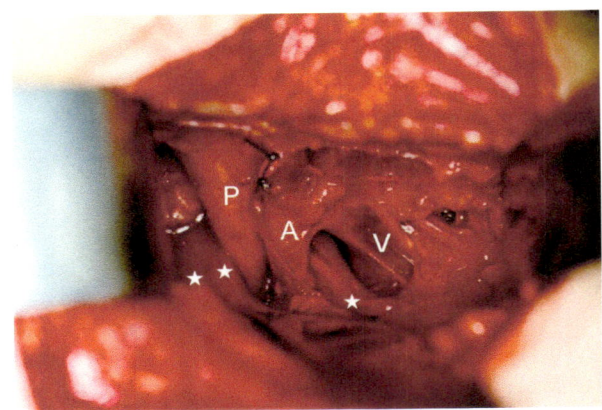

Fig. 5.29 Intraoperative presentation of median scalene muscle, curved forceps below (*2 asterisks*). Anterior scalene muscle already loosened (*asterisk*). *P* brachial plexus, *A* subclavian artery. (From Wilhelm and Wilhelm 1985, with kind permission from Thieme)

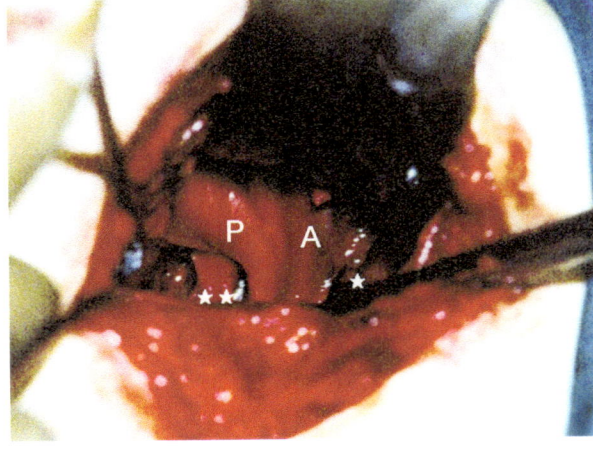

intercostal muscles from the lower rim of the 1st rib, it is loosened in posterior and anterior direction with a rib raspatory. Resection of the rib is accomplished by using a rib forceps and a Luer retractor elbowed at the handle, in order to have a good view of the surgical site. Together with the plexus root retractor promoted by Roos, this instrument is perfectly suited, especially if the trough-shaped end piece is not flexed, lengthening the direction of the instrument's shaft. Both lower plexus roots can be directly retracted from the inner rim of the 1st rib, and resection of the rib in the posterior area, according to Roos, approximately 1 cm distal to the thoracic vertebra transverse process can be performed.

The author, however, performs rib resection up to the costovertebral joint if anatomic topographic conditions allow for it, in order to prevent a possible irritation of the lower plexus roots by the stump of the rib, especially in reverse motion of the arm.

The place of resection has to be even, and possible bone peaks have to be removed by Luer, as they can lead to arm plexus and pleural injury. Anterior parts of the rib are resected at the rib cartilage; if the remaining stump of the rib should still irritate the subclavian vein, it can also be removed by exarticulation in the sternocostal joint.

Presentation of the cupula pleurae and possibly a pleurovertebral ligament, which is resected (Fig. 5.26), follows after resection of the 1st rib. The cupula pleurae is loosened and exposed without cutting, and then the posterior wall of the subclavian vein and the internal thoracic artery and the phrenic nerve are prepared resecting the compressing Sibson fascia, which can contain all anatomic structures, mentioned (Fig. 5.30).

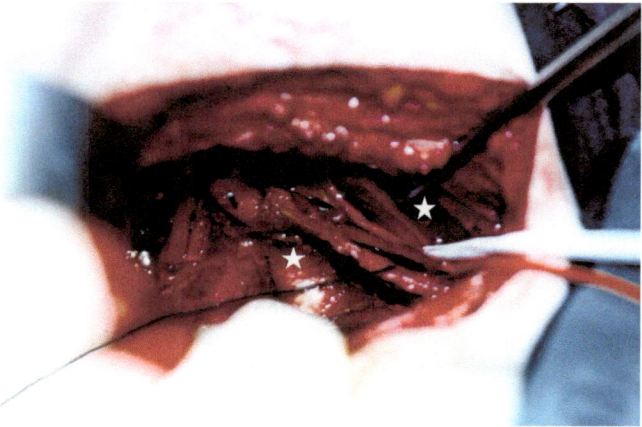

Fig. 5.30 Status post decompression of right nerve-vessel strand by resection of 1st rib, desinsertion of anterior and median scalene muscles and resection of subclavian muscle. Defect of this muscle on right side of picture marked by *asterisk*. White snare: phrenic nerve; red snare: internal thoracic artery; black snare: strong fibromuscular structure, including a disturbing subclavian artery, not dissected yet. *Left asterisk*: right brachiocephalic trunk with subclavian artery, well recognisable due to ligature of the superior thoracic artery origin. Brachial plexus on left side of picture. (From Wilhelm and Wilhelm 1985, with kind permission from Thieme)

Preoperatively these structures might be seen phlebographically in the shape of a striped vertical impression (Fig. 5.12).

After decompression of the subclavian vein, the resection of the upper thoracic sympathetic nerve follows with removal of the three proximal ganglia, the first of which frequently melts with the inferior cervical ganglion into the stellate ganglion (Fig. 5.3). If anatomic conditions are difficult, this resection can also be replaced by neurotomy of the communicating branches leading to the lower plexus roots (Rieder 1933).

Fine clips may be placed in adjacent tissue in order to mark the resection area; however, they must not be placed at the sympathetic stumps, leading to an increase in *postsympathectomy pain*, or even causing it. Then haemorrhage and wound conditions are controlled at the cupula pleurae. Small pleural lesions are harmless and do not need to be treated. Larger lesions are sewn. *If there is injury of the pleural cupula, a water check is recommended.* After preparation of the lesion, wound closure follows by atraumatic suture with final repetition of the water check. If there are pleural lesions which cannot be closed completely, only adapting sutures are made and a Redon drainage size 14 is inserted into the pleural space with sufficient perforations for drainage of wound fluid in the axillary area. After wound closure layer by layer finishing with intracutaneous skin suture, and application of a simple adhesive dressing, a postoperative lung x-ray should be done if the peak of the lung was injured and also in the case of bleeding to rule out a pneumo- or a haematothorax.

5.9   Postoperative Treatment (Fig. 5.31)

Postoperatively the patient is placed with slightly elevated upper body and simultaneous arm abduction in intermediate position. A pasted stockinette is helpful for hanging the forearm.

Permanent individual pain therapy is continued postoperatively with dosage adaptation. A survey of possible medication is shown in Table 5.7 staged according to WHO standard (modified according to Wilhelm 2011).

Professional help should accompany patients with low blood pressure when getting out of bed, walking on the healthy side, in order not to catch the operated arm in a reflex if the patient collapses, jeopardising the brachial plexus by possible traction damage (Table 5.11, patient 20). When getting out of bed, the patient should also always receive its preordered abduction dressing in order to prevent pain-triggering motion in the shoulder joint and traction stress of the brachial plexus. Also keep in mind a dressing always conveys the signal of "noli me tangere/do not touch".

Drainage is only removed after completion of wound secretion. An x-ray on the 3rd day is recommended to rule out haemorrhage. In case there is a haematoma in the depth of the wound, it has to be removed and drained immediately to prevent irritating and compressing scarring in the armpit. Sutures are removed no earlier than 10 days after surgery.

Cautious active motion exercises are postoperatively only performed with the fingers and the propped-up elbow joint as far as the patient complies according to

Surgical procedure	Therapeutic effect
A. Decompression of subclavian vein (removal of stenosis)	1. Improvement of venous back-flow 2. Vanishing of peripheral edema 3. Reduction of subfascial pressure 4. Improvement of microcirculation, perfusion of tissue and cell metabolism
B. Decompression of subclavian artery	Reduction of sympathetic efferences
C. Decompression of plexus roots (C8 and Th 1)	1. Reduction of sympathetic efferences 2. Improvement of influence of mechanoceptive, pain-inhibiting afferences (A β-fibrous)
D. Transaxillary sympathectomy	1. Discontinuation of main strand of sympathetic efferences 2. Reduction of sweat secretion 3. Reduction of peripheral vessel resistance 4. Improvement of metabolism 5. Reduction of algogenous substances 6. Reduction of painful afferences (A δ-and C-fibres)

Improvement of pain-inhibitory and pain-conducting function of spinal cord posterior horn synapses

Fig. 5.31 Surgical treatment of CRPS I. (From Wilhelm 1997b)

his pain limit and under surveillance of his physician. *Any passive motion therapy of the operated arm is forbidden*!

- *Manual passive therapeutic hand treatment first is only allowed on the healthy side, for instance, lymphatic drainage and cautious extension treatment of the finger and hand joints.*

This treatment should be accompanied by connective tissue and fascia techniques and a corresponding training for sensibility as well. Here "this training is confronted with the mobility problem being basis for the recovery of fine myokinetic function and the entire conception of the operated arm" (Tenyèr 2002).

"This treatment should first be performed as vibration therapy which then can be completed by treatment with hard brushes, spiked ball etc. (movable triggers, effect via reflex path). Only then therapy with soft brushes, paint brushes and in shape of static stimuli (tuning fork, wooden- and metal pins, smooth and raw surfaces should follow" (Tenyèr 2002).

Table 5.7 CRPS I: treatment of postoperative pain (examples)

	WHO-stage I for level "good" non-opioids	WHO-stage II for level "fair" mild opioids	WHO-stage III for level "insufficient" strong opioids
Medication	Acetylsalicylic acid	Codeine (Gelon.®Paintab.)	Morphine
	Diclofenac	Tilidine-N (Valoron ret.®)	Buprenorphine
	Ibuprofen	Tramadol	Morphine ret.
	Novamin	Codeine ret.	Oxycodone ret.
	Paracetamol	Tilidine-N ret.	Hydromorphone ret.
		Tramadol ret.	Fentanyl plaster
Adjuvants	Corticoids	Amitriptyline	Ganglion
	Gabapentin (Neurontin®)	Valium®	Stellate block
	Katadolon		Plexus anaesthesia
	Tolperison (Mydocalm®)		(With naropin®)
	Biphosphonate		Continuous plexus anaesthesia

Medication supplemented and modified according to Wilhelm (2011)

"It is known, this therapy also reflects on the operated arm as a consensual reaction, depending on the extent of the pre-operative pain improvement; this therapy can also be started at the operated arm after 3–4 weeks, *whereby pain-afferences caused by treatment have to be prevented in any case*. Problems and deterioration of local findings in the further course of therapy have to be discussed with the surgeon" (Tenyèr 2002).

This disease sometimes is a big problem for hand therapists, as they are afraid of hand stiffness, sometimes therapeutically leading to hasty actions. This in the course of time results in a progressive deterioration of functional findings and the pain values reached by surgery with a corresponding "final result", as shown in follow-up examinations (Table 5.11, pat. 11, 17 and 18).

There is a very depressing course of a female patient still needing treatment, who was passively treated for over 2 years by flexing the hand over the table border and by passively flexing the fingers in order to accomplish fist closure; this unfortunately is not a single case!

Force in the treatment of CRPS I, as well as in its postoperative course, can only reach negative results! On the contrary sensibility and renouncing of all measures leading to damage of pain afferences, as well as an individual, cautious, quiet and calm treatment of the patient is asked for. Figures 5.32, 5.33, 5.34 and 5.35 show how unnecessary and harmful any passive action can be. They demonstrate an edematous hand stiffened in extension for 2 years, showing a full extension and a nearly complete flexion in the MP joints of the fingers in the afternoon of the day of surgery. At this point the distinct edema had almost completely vanished as well, and development of skin folds over the joints was completely developed again. Similar direct postoperative improvement in diverse extent was also seen in the remaining good results (Tables 5.10 and 5.11).

Fig. 5.32 Preoperative function of a severe CRPS I of the left hand after 2 years of conservative therapy. Due to the resistant edema, the crease above the MP and IP joints is not visible any more (patient 19, Table 5.11)

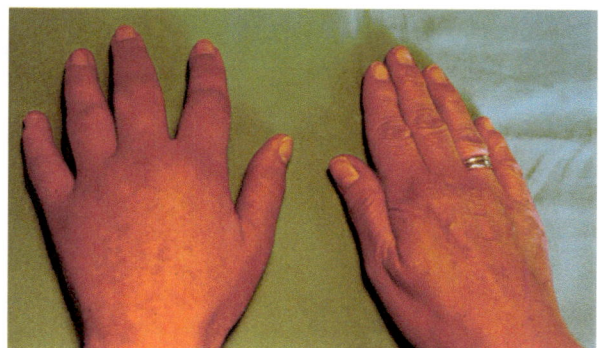

Fig. 5.33 Preoperative picture of pathologic hand from the side shows a significant extension stiffness of all fingers

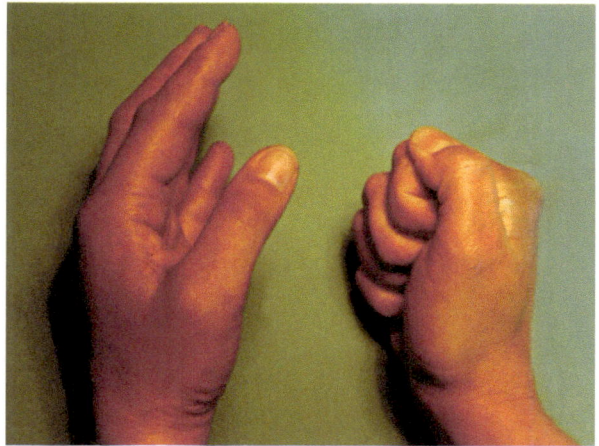

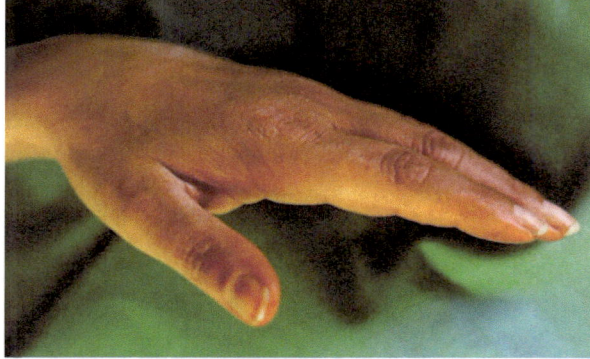

Fig. 5.34 Postoperatively in the afternoon of the day of surgery, there is a free finger extension and a complete reconstitution of skin folds above the joints mentioned

Fig. 5.35 Postoperatively there is a quite complete flexion in the MP joints and a fingertip-palm of hand distance of 5 cm

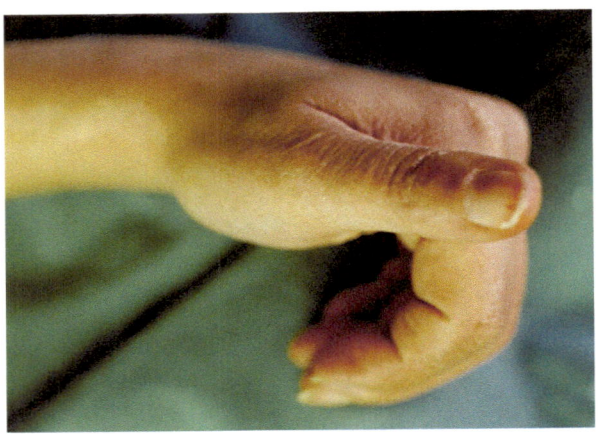

5.10   Results

In order to judge the transaxillary procedure used, the picture series of 4 patients were presented first (19, 7, 4 and 8) (patient 19: Figs. 5.32, 5.33, 5.34 and 5.35; patient 7: Figs. 5.36 and 5.37; patient 4: Figs. 5.38, 5.39 and 5.40; patient 8: Figs. 5.41 and 5.42).

Between 1984 and 1991 ten patients were treated surgically after an average pretreatment time of 9 months, and postoperative results were excellent in 70 %, good in 20 % and fair in 10 %.

Postoperative treatment with *Valoron N* was only necessary in three out of ten patients (Table 5.10, patient 2, 8 and 9). Further on only antiphlogistics, psychopharmacologic agents, neurobion and regular pain medication, like paracetamol, were given.

Complications only were a pneumothorax, which was drained, and a postoperative haemorrhage from the intercostal artery I, which had to be reoperated.

An unexpected deterioration of the examination results and the pain score was found in a female patient after completion of treatment, and after starting the working process again, in this case an implantation of a "spinal cord stimulator" had to be undertaken (Table 5.10, patient 9).

In patients treated between 2000 and 2002 (Table 5.11), it was found quite early that not all of the ten patients with a longer preoperative treatment showed fair results, especially patient 11, whereas patient 17 initially showed a good result, but in the further course had a deterioration of findings due to her own fault, that is, by non-compliance concerning the treatment agreed upon prior to surgery, finally resulting in complete therapy resistance. The more striking result was found in patient 13, who was only surgically treated after over 12 years of pretreatment. Postoperative result ranges between 3 and 4, mainly based on a very painful intercostal neuralgia. In this case a neurotomy of intercostal nerves in two sessions resulted in significant improvement.

Fig. 5.36 These pictures show a massive hand and forearm edema in CRPS I after surgery of a massive palm of the hand phlegmone and the reconstitution of edema after 4 days. Due to a severe subclavian vein stenosis (Fig. 5.16), the patient was already surgically treated after 2 months. Postoperative treatment was completed after only 6 months (patient 7) (From Wilhelm 1997b)

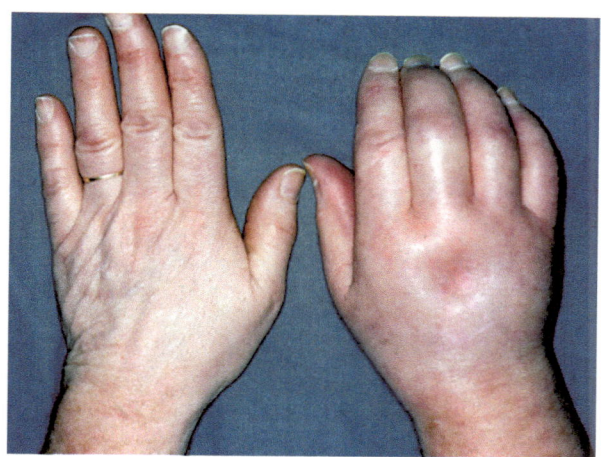

Fig. 5.37 Edema vanished in 4 days. Postoperative result cf. Table 5.9 and 5.10 (From Wilhelm 1997b)

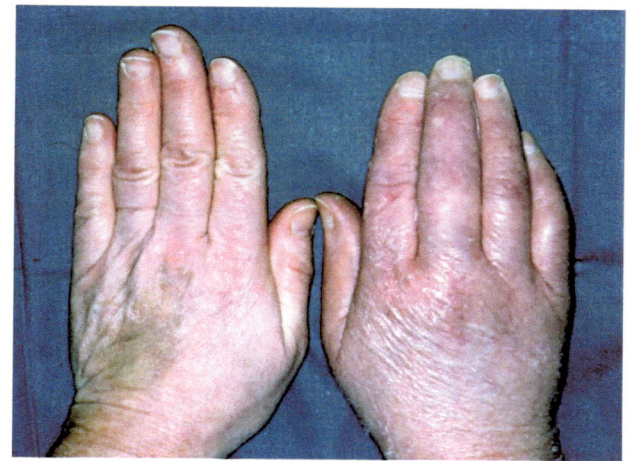

In judging these results, the still in some cases insufficient primary pain medication as well as the passive motion therapy has to be taken into account as causal aspects. Also the time of diagnosis and the start of adequate treatment have to be considered.

In group 3 complications were narrow mantle pneumothorax requiring treatment. An increasing pneumothorax after stellate blockade had to be treated by thoracic drainage, however.

Table 5.12 presents the procedures for the treatment of therapy-resistant Sudeck's dystrophy (CRPS I), performed in Germany and England. Successful results were reached in 44 (84.61 %) out of 52 cases; thus, *this surgical technique can be commonly recommended as standard procedure.*

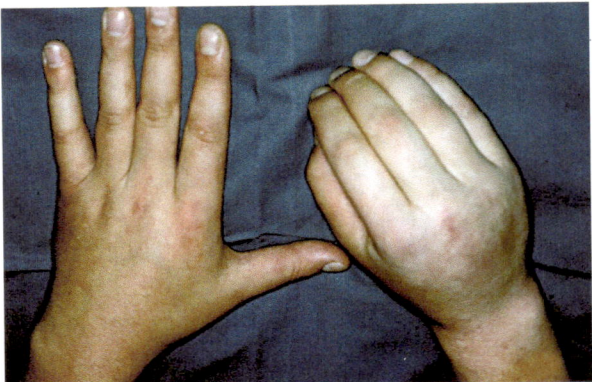

Fig. 5.38 CRPS I in a "non-thrombotic obstruction" of right subclavian vein (patient 4, Fig. 5.18). Edema is limited to the hand due to excellent collateral circle. Even the smallest attempt at motion results in severe pain, *VAS level in rest* 8–10. The hand is completely "stiffened" in flexion and adduction of fingers. After 2 months of postoperative treatment, the patient was free of pain and was able to completely extend his fingers and close his fist. (From Wilhelm 1997b)

Fig. 5.39 Free extension of fingers 2 months after surgery, significant atrophy of soft tissue at the hand

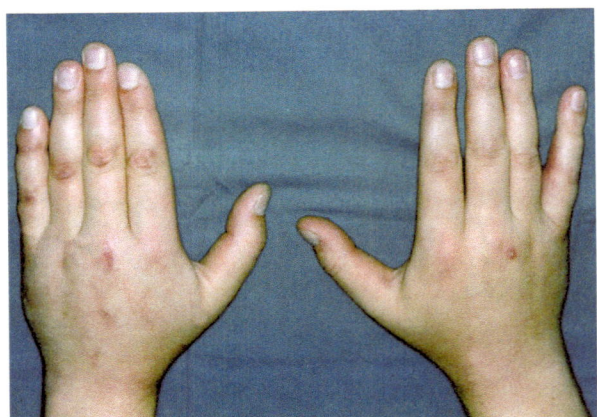

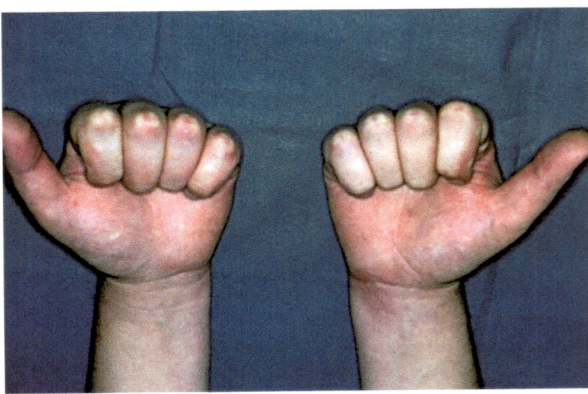

Fig. 5.40 Complete fist closure of fingers, significant atrophy of soft tissue in the forearm

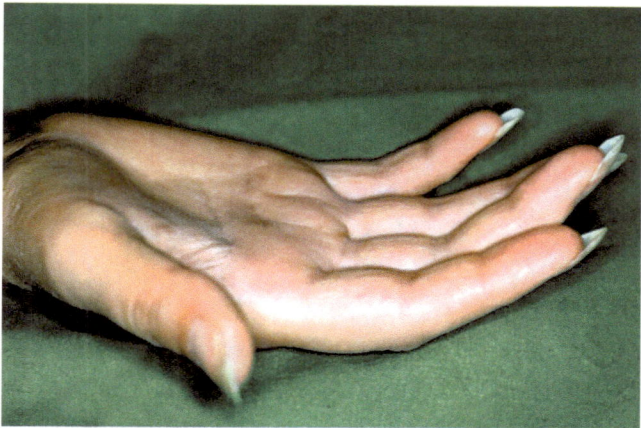

Fig. 5.41 CRPS I after conservative therapy for 11 months (patient 8). Indication for surgery due to significant pain, inhibition of finger extension and lack of crude strength. After postoperative treatment for 5 months, the patient was free of pain

Fig. 5.42 This patient also showed a significant inhibition of fist closure (postoperative function Tables 5.9 and 5 10)

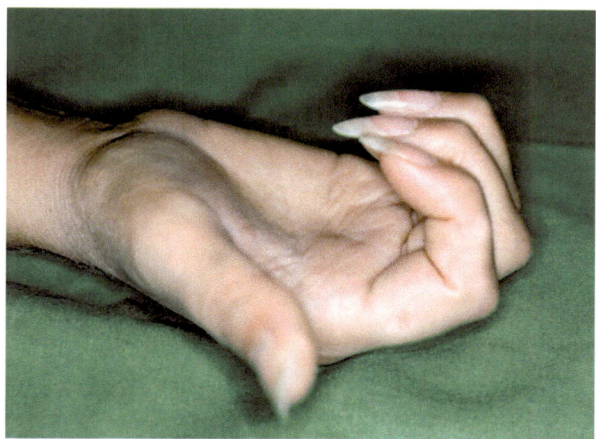

The author performed this procedure in 26 patients, and 6 patients were not taken into account, however, as treatment has not been concluded, yet. Further operations were done in Germany and England.

The causal aspects for explaining different surgical results in group II mentioned in the prior section do not suffice to answer all corresponding questions. This is mainly true for patient 13, where a much worse surgical result was expected, knowing about the ongoing stress of the pain inhibitory system of the dorsal horn of the spinal cord for years, whereas in patient 17 a much more positive result was expected due to the shorter pretreatment time, in spite of the fact he did not comply with the postoperative treatment course, exclusively due to occupational reasons.

Table 5.8 CRPS I: evaluation of results

Result	Grip strength (%)	Flexion deficit (cm)	Extension deficit (cm)	Pain VAS values	Evaluation
Excellent	>50	0–1	0–2	0–(1)[a]	None
Good	30–50	–2	–3	1–(3)[a]	Minimal
Fair	10–30	–4	–4	3–(6)[a]	Slight
Poor	<10	Unchanged	Unchanged	6–10	Insufficient

[a]Maximum pain level under severe stress

Table 5.9 CRPS I (1984–1991): reconstitution of strength and function of finger

Patient no.	Grip strength (%)	Flexion deficit — Preoperative / Postoperative	Extension deficit — Preoperative / Postoperative	Follow-up period (years)
1	68.8	$\dfrac{3-3.5-3-2.5}{0-0-0-0.5}$	$\dfrac{6-6-5-4}{0-0-0-0}$	10
2	77.1	$\dfrac{3-2-2-2.5}{0-0-0-0}$	$\dfrac{5-6-5-3.5}{0-0-0-0}$	9
3	60.0	$\dfrac{3.5\ \ 3\ \ 2\ \ 1.5}{1\ \ 0.5\ \ 0\ \ 0}$	$\dfrac{4.5\ \ 3.5\ \ 2\ \ 2}{0\ \ 1\ \ 2\ \ 0}$	9
4	98.0	$\dfrac{5-5-5-5.5}{0-0-0-0}$	$\dfrac{7-7.5-7-6}{0-0-0-0}$	9
5	48.7	$\dfrac{5-4.5-3-2.5}{0.5-0-0-0}$	$\dfrac{2-3-3-1.5}{1-1-1-1.5}$	8
6	93.1	$\dfrac{4.5\ \ 5\ \ 5\ \ 4.5}{0\ \ 0\ \ 0\ \ 0}$	$\dfrac{1-2.5-2.5-3.5}{0.5-0-0-1}$	7
7	40.4	$\dfrac{4-4.5-5-5}{1-2-3.5-3}$	$\dfrac{4-5-4.5-4}{0-1.5-2-3.5^a}$	7
8	82.8	$\dfrac{3.5\ \ 3\ \ 3\ \ 2.5}{0\ \ 0\ \ 0\ \ 0}$	$\dfrac{3-4-2.5-3.5}{0-0-0-0}$	5
9	17.9	$\dfrac{7-10.5-9.5-8.5}{1.5-2.5-2-1.5}$	$\dfrac{4.5\ \ 2\ \ 2\ \ 1.5}{0\ \ 0\ \ 1\ \ 0}$	4
10	17.0	$\dfrac{8.5\ \ 9\ \ 8\ \ 7}{4\ \ 3.5\ \ 4\ \ 3}$	$\dfrac{1.5\ \ 3\ \ 2\ \ 1.5}{0\ \ 2.5\ \ 2.5\ \ 0^b}$	7

From Wilhelm (1997a, b)
[a]Status following operation of palmar phlegmon
[b]Status following operation of tendon and nerve injury

Table 5.10 CRPS I: surgical results (1984–1991)

Patient no.	Duration of treatment (months)			Postoperative results		
	Preoperative	Postoperative	Total	Pain[a]	Horner S.	Evaluation
1	14	9	3	–	–	Excellent
2	8	6	14	–	–	Excellent
3	11	9	20	–	((+))	Excellent
4	7	2	9	–	((+))	Excellent
5	19	1	20	–	–	Excellent
6	3	4	7	–	–	Excellent
7	2	6	8	–	–	Good
8	11	5	16	–	–	Excellent
9	7	42	49	((+))	((+))	Fair
10	9	9	18	((+))	–	Good
Average:	9	9	18 (months)			

From Wilhelm (1997a, b)
Follow-up $\varnothing$ 7.5 (4–10) years
Results: 7×excellent=70 %, 2×good=20 %, 1×fair=10 %
[a]Evaluation of pain (VAS)

5.11 Pain Inhibitory Function of Dorsal Horn Synapsis System

In this situation it was a lucky coincidence the author attended a presentation of Zieglgänzberger, Max Planck Institute, Munich in 2004, where he was shown results of an animal experiment, which can prove the increase of strength and frequency of pain afferences after a sufficient duration of time leads to a destruction of the cell core of the interneuron via excessive run-in of calcium ions by associated processes, thus resulting in a loss of pain inhibitory function of the dorsal horn synapsis system.

As this experiment also scientifically proves the results of a contraindicated passive physiotherapy in CRPS I, the functions of the inhibitory dorsal horn synapsis system under normal and pathologic conditions are shortly presented.

In relaxation the glutamate necessary for neurotransmission is accumulated in the presynaptic neuron, and the calcium channel associated with the N-Methyl-D-ASPARTATE (NMDA) receptor of the postsynaptic neuron (interneuron) of the dorsal horn synapsis system is occluded by magnesium ions. At this time the concentration of intracellular calcium in the postsynaptic neuron is low (Fig. 5.43).

At the same time in severe and ongoing pain, substance P can be released.

In order to end the magnesium blockade, the receptor needs to be activated by ligands, in this case by the glutamate released in the intracellular gap, and the postsynaptic neuron needs to be depolarized. It is important that even minor depolarization of the cellular membrane due to the relatively poor binding qualities of the magnesium loosens the blockade of the ion channel for the run-in of calcium into the cell of the postsynaptic neuron (Fig. 5.44).

Table 5.11   CRPS I: surgical results (2000–2008/2002)

Patient no.	Treatment duration (months)			Postoperative results			Findings	
	Preoperative	Postoperative	Total	Pain	Horner	1–4[a]	Preoperative	Intraoperative
11	21	24 →	45	(+)	+	4	a +, b 160°	d2
12	35	19 →	54	(+)	−	1	a +, b 160°	d2
13	148	19 →	167	((+))	(+)	2	a +, b 50°	d3
14	28	6 →	34	−	((+))	1	a ((+)), —	d3
15	28	13 →	51	((+))	((+))	2	a +, b 70°	c2
16	18	1 →	19	−	((+))	1	a (+), —	c1*
17	13	10 →	23	(+) →	++	4	a ++, b 20°	c1*
18	76	8 →	84	(+)	(+)	3	a +, b 30°	c2
19	27	3 →	30	((+))	((+))	1	a ((+)), b 80°	c2
20	22	7 →	29	(+) → +	(+)	2 (4[b])	a +, b 160°	c3
Average	43	11	54 (months)			Results: excellent = 40 %; good = 30 %; fair = 10 %; insufficient = 20 %		
Average	(30)	(10)	(41) (months)[c]					

From Wilhelm (1997a, b)

a preoperative shoulder symptomatology [((+)) — ++], *b* preoperative shoulder contraction, *c* sympathicoresection; number of ganglia, *d* neurotomy of post-ganglionic branches, number, ++ remarkably long ganglion

[a]Evaluation: 1–4

[b](Patient 20): s/p severe traction damage of right brachial plexus on 2nd postoperative day due to external influence. Hand function not utilisable

[c]Postoperative results after extrapolation of Pat. No. 13

Table 5.12 Surgical treatment of resistant CRPS I:collective statistics (1984–2002)

Hospital	No. of cases	Results	
Aschaffenburg Teaching Hospital Department of Surgery (own cases 1984–2002)	20((+6)[a]	11×	Excellent
		5×	Good
		2×	Fair
		2×	Insufficient
Diakonisse Hospital Kassel Department of Vescular Surgery	4	4×	Successful[b]
Aachen University Surgery Department of Plastic and Reconstructive Surgery	1	1×	Excellent[c]
Bradford Teaching Hospital Dpt. Trauma/ Orthopaedics Bradford BD 9 6RJ (1994–2006)	27 (+2)[d]	17×	Excellent and good[d]
		4×	Fair
		6×	Insufficient
Total	52 (+8)[a]	44×	Successful

From Wilhelm (2007)
[a]Postoperative treatment of 6 patients not completed yet
[b]Personal information of Prof. Dr. J.D. Gruß
[c]Result of own follow-up
[d]Personal information of R. Boome, MD. (2006) – 2 patients not taken into account

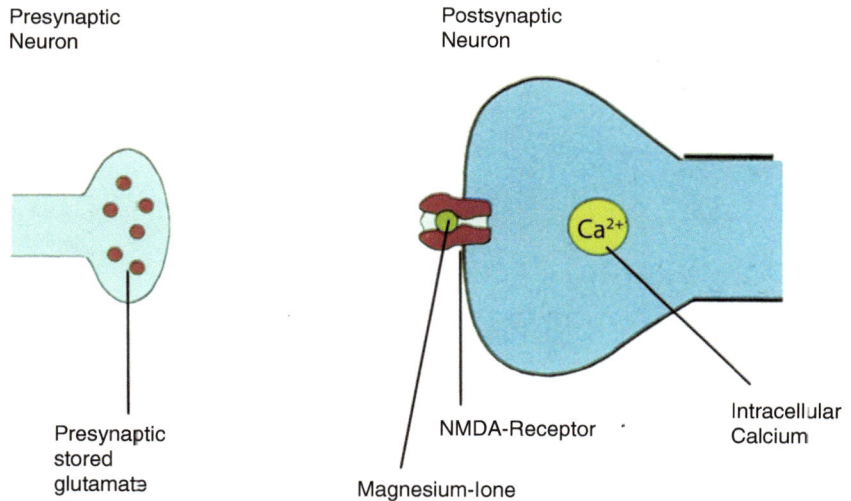

Presynaptic Neuron

Postsynaptic Neuron

Presynaptic stored glutamate

Magnesium-Ione

NMDA-Receptor

Intracellular Calcium

Fig. 5.43 Schematic presentation of functional entity at a glutamate synapsis. (With kind permission of Merz 2003)

In pathologic conditions, for instance, in increase of frequency and strength of pain afferences, the release and absorption of glutamate is less controlled. Thus, the concentration of glutamate in the synaptic gap rises only slightly. If this happens over a longer stretch of time, however, the amount of glutamate reached suffices to stop the magnesium blockade of the calcium channel with calcium ions permanently entering the postsynaptic neuron (interneuron), finally leading to a pathologic increase of intercellular calcium level initiating degeneration of the interneuron in the course of time (Fig. 5.45).

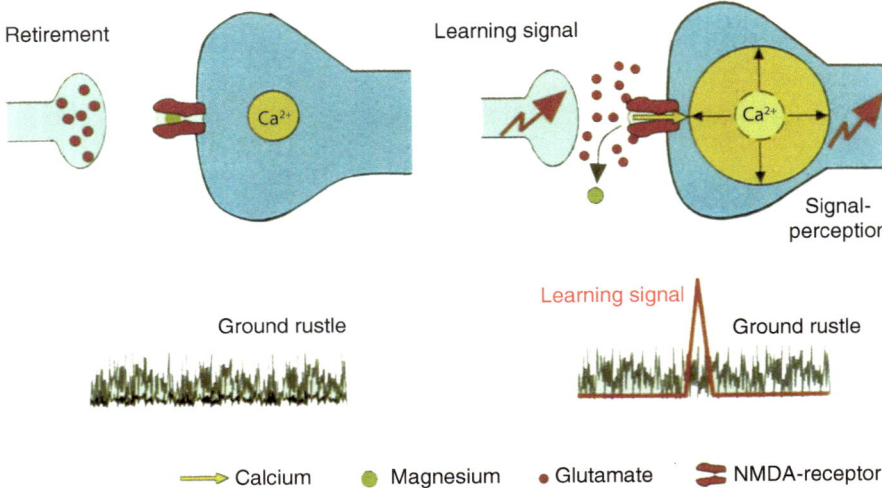

Fig. 5.44 Regular glutamate triggered neurotransmission at NMDA receptor. (With kind permission from Merz 2003)

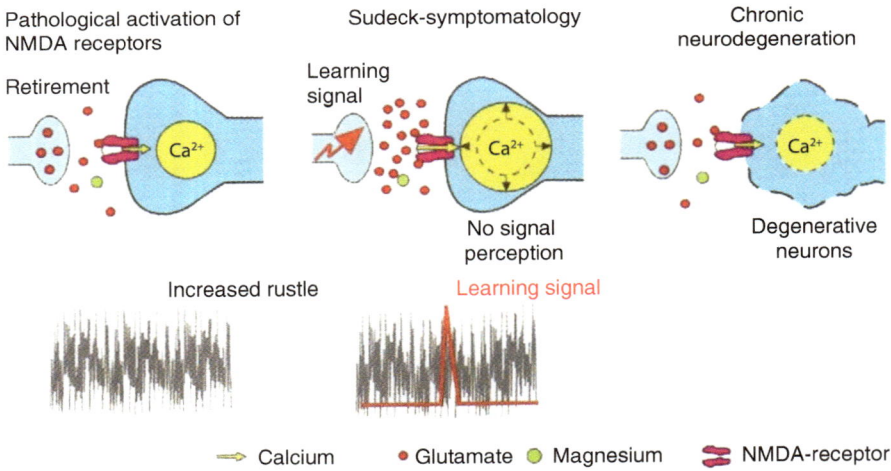

Fig. 5.45 Disturbed glutamate neurotransmission with clinical and neurogenous results. DAT symptoms replaced by CRPS I symptoms. (With kind permission from Merz 2003)

"Memantine" (AXURA), originally produced by Merz company for the treatment of Alzheimer's disease, physiologically works like magnesium, further on being able to block the NMDA receptor in the synaptic gap even in the presence persistent pathologic concentrations of glutamate due to its much better binding qualities, protecting the poststenotic neuron from the pathologic run-in of calcium triggered by glutamate (neuroprotective effect; Fig. 5.46).

Under normal conditions memantine does not have a negative influence on the flow in of calcium ions.

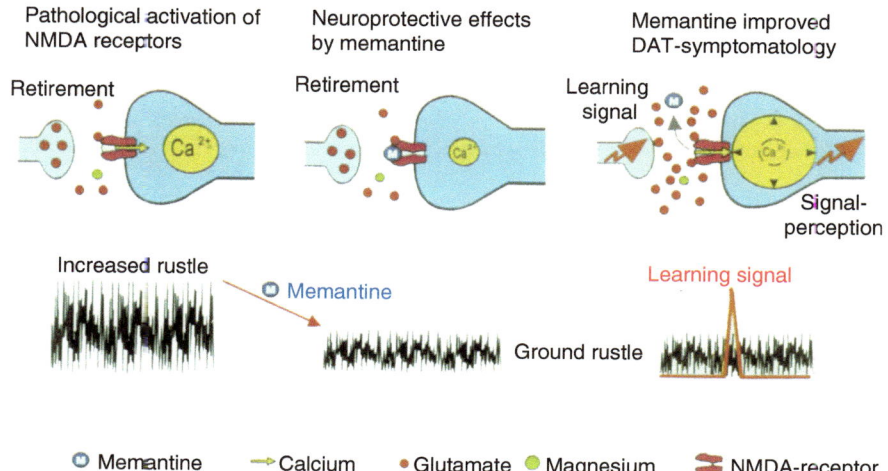

Fig. 5.46 Mechanism of NMDA receptor antagonist memantine which can improve Alzheimer-dementia (DAT) as well as CRPS I symptoms at an early stage. (With kind permission from Merz 2003)

This short synopsis of the glutamate neurotransmission in the product monography of AXURA by Merz company/Frankfurt is by no means complete. It should only draw attention of the interested reader towards the functional problem of the pain-inhibiting system of the dorsal horn of the spinal cord in Sudeck's dystrophy, serving as scientific proof for all therapists of the dramatically negative influence of additionally triggered pain afferences, especially in passive motion exercise in the treatment of CRPS I.

5.12 Mistakes, Dangers and Complications

The possibility of injuring the lower plexus roots is relatively less in an experienced surgeon. Haemorrhage from the intercostal artery I and small venous vessels cannot always be prevented. Frequently there are pleural lesions, whereas injuries at the pleural cupula are rare, and they only occur in attempts at suture of a pleural tear.

References

Baron R, Zieglgänsberger W (o. J.) Neuropathischer Schmerz (CD-Rom) [Neuropathic pain]. Pfizer, Pain

Bär E, Felder M, Kiener B (Hrsg) (2002) Algodystrophy (Complex regional pain syndrome I). SUVA – Novartis, 2. Auflage, S 11–14, S 18–20. Siehe im Internet unter www.suva.ch, Bestell-Nr. 2771.d.

Bircher JL (1981) Schmerzsyndrome [Pain syndromes]. In: Nigst H, Buck-Gramcko D, Milesi H (Hrsg) (eds) Handchirurgie, Band 1. Thieme, Stuttgart/New York

Blumberg H, Hoffmann U (1994) Zur Diagnostik der sympathischen Reflexdystrophie [Diagnostics of sympathetic reflex dystrophy]. Nervenarzt 65:370–374

Blumensaat C (1956) Der heutige Stand der Lehre vom Sudeck-Syndrom [Today's situation of teaching on Sudeck's syndrome]. Hefte Unfallheilk 51:1–225

Boome R, Iha KN, Kittopp K (2006) Surgical treatment of complex regional pain syndrome type I by subclavian vein release (persönliche Mitteilung, in preparation)

Dunant JH (ed) (1987) Das neurovaskuläre Schultergürtelsyndrom – Thoracic outlet-Syndrom [The neurovascular shoulder girdle syndrome – the thoracic-outlet-syndrome], 2. Aufl. Huber, Bern

Ehlert H (1974) Neue Gesichtspunkte zur Genese des Sudeck-Syndroms [New aspects on Sudecks syndrome genesis]. Mschr Unfallheilk 77:417–421

Grünert J (1993) Untersuchungen zur Pathophysiologie des Morbus Sudeck [Research on pathophysiology of Morbus Sudeck]. Habilitationsschrift der Westfälischen Wilhelmsuniversität zu Münster

Hackethal KH (1958) Das Sudeck'sche Syndrom [Sudeck's syndrome]. In: Schaefer HC (ed) Medizin, Theorie und Klinik. Hüthig, Frankfurt

Hannington-Kiff JG (1977) Relief of Sudeck's atrophy by regional intravenous guanethidine. Lancet 28:1132

Lankford LL (1993) Reflex sympathetic dystrophy. In: Green DP (Hrsg) Operative handsurgery, 3. Aufl. Livingstone, New York, pp S627–S660

Leriche R (1923) Sur les dés equilibres vaso-moteurs post, traumatiques primitifs des extrémités [On basic posttraumatic vasculomotor balance of extremities]. Lyon Chir 20:746–753

Merz (2003) Wissenschaftliche Produktmonografie AXURA [Scientific product monography of Axura], Frankfurt

Mitchel SW, Morehouse G, Keen WW (1864) Gunshot wounds and other injuries of nerves. Lippincott, Philadelphia

Rieder W (1933) Resektion der zur Hand gehenden Rr. Communicantes [Resection of communicating branches leading towards the hand]. Chirurg 5:219–224

Roos DB (1977) Transaxillary extrapleural thoracic sympathectomy. In: Surgical techniques illustrated, vol 2. Little, Brown & Co, Boston

Schink W (1972) Vasomotorische und trophische Störungen [Vasculomotor and trophic disturbances]. In: Wachsmuth W, Wilhelm A (Hrsg) Die Operationen an der Hand, Band X, Teil 3 der Allgemeinen und speziellen chirurgische Operationslehre. Springer, Heidelberg, pp S429–440

Sinis N, Bibaumer N, Schwarz A, Unertl K, Schaller HE, Haerle M (2006) Memantine und komplexes regionales Schmerzsyndrom (CRPS): Behandlungseffekte und kortikale Reorganisation [Memantine and complex regional pain syndrome (CRPS): effects of treatment and cortical reorganisation]. Handchir Mikrochir Plast Chir 38:164–171

Sudeck P (1900) Ueber die acute entzündliche Knochenatrophie [On acute inflammatory bone atrophy]. Langenbecks Arch Klin Chir 62:147–156

Sudeck P (1902) Ueber die acute (trophoneurotische) Knochenatrophie nach Entzündungen und Traumen der Extremitäten [On acute (trophoneurotic) bone atrophy after inflammations and trauma of the extremities] Dtsch Med Wschr 28:336–338

Sudeck P (1931) Die trophische Extremitätenstörung durch periphere (infektiöse und traumatische) Reize [Trophic Extremity Disturbance by Peripheral (Infectious and Traumatic) Irritation] Dtsch Med Wschr 234:596–602

Sudman E, Sundsfjord JA (1984) Relief from pain in Sudeck's posttraumatic syndrome by fasciotomy. Arch Orthop Trauma Surg 103:185–189

Tenyér M (2002) Zusammenfassung der Erfahrungen der Patienten aus der M. Sudeck-Selbsthilfegruppe "Sympathische Hände" in Berlin [Summary of patient experience in the Sudeck's self- help group 'sympathetic hands' in Berlin. Z Handther 5:18–19

von Lanz T, Wachsmuth W (eds) (1955) Praktische Anatomie [Practical anatomy], Band I, Teil 2, Hals. Springer, Berlin

von Lanz T, Wachsmuth W (Hrsg) (1959) Praktische Anatomie [Practical anatomy], Band I, Teil 3, Arm, 2. Aufl. Springer, Berlin

Werner CO (1979) Lateral elbow pain and posterior interosseous nerve entrapment. Acta Orthop Scand Suppl II 174:1–62

Wilhelm A (1958) Die Innervation der Gelenke der oberen Extremität [Articular innervation of the upper extremity]. Z Anat Entwickl Gesch 120:331–371

Wilhelm A (1972) Die gezielte Schmerzausschaltung am Schultergelenk [Aimed pain elimination at the shoulder joint]. In: Wachsmuth W, Wilhelm A (Hrsg) Die Operationen an der Hand. Band X, Teil 3 Der Allgemeinen und Speziellen Chirurgischen Operationslehre. Springer, Berlin/Heidelberg/New York, pp S50–S54

Wilhelm A (1997a) Stenosis of the subclavian vein. An unknown cause of resistant reflex sympathetic dystrophy. Hand Clin 13:387–411

Wilhelm A (1997b) Operative Behandlung der therapieresistenten Sudeck'schen Dystrophie durch transaxilläre Dekompression des Nervengefäßstranges und Sympathektomie [Surgical treatment of therapy resistant Sudeck's dystrophy by transaxillary decompression of the nerve- vessel- bundle and sympathectomy]. Zur Pathogenese des M. Sudeck. Handchir Mikrochir Plast Chir 29:60–72

Wilhelm A (2007) Neue Aspekte der Behandlung von therapieresistenten Sudeck'schen Dystrophien [New aspects on the treatment of therapy resistant Sudeck's dystrophy]. Vortrag, gehalten am 14.04. auf dem 4. Polnisch-Deutschen Symposium in Stettin (Szczeciw)

Wilhelm A (2011) Die operative Behandlung der therapieresistenten Sudeck-Dystrophie (CRPS I) durch transaxilläre Dekompression des Nerven-Gefäß-Stranges und obere extrapleurale thorakale Sympathikusresektion [Surgical technique of transaxillary decompression of neurovascular bundle and extrapleurale resection of upper sympathetic trunc, respectively neurotomy of communicating branches running towards the lower plexus roots] In: Towfigh H et al. (eds) Hand Surgery, Volume 1. Springer-Verlag Berlin Heidelberg, pp 438–465.

Wilhelm A, Englert D (1989) Die Bedeutung der V. subclavia-Stenose für die Behandlung der Dupuytren'schen Kontraktur [The significance of the subclavian vein stenosis for treatment of Dupuytren's contracture]. Handchir Mikrochir Plast Chir 21:66–71

Wilhelm A, Wilhelm F (1985) Das Thoracic outlet-Syndrom und seine Bedeutung für die Chirurgie der Hand [The thoracic-outlet-syndrome and its significance for hand surgery]. Handchir Mikrochir Plast Chir 17:173–187

Winkel R, Blonder A (2011) Therapie chronischer Schmerzen und des komplexen regionalen Schmerzsyncroms (CRPS I) [Therapy of chronic pains and of the complex regional pain-syndroms (CRPS I)]. In Towfigh H et al. (2011) Handsurgery Volume I. Page 399–421. Springer-Verlag Berlin Heidelberg 2011.

Zimmermann M, Handwerker HO (eds) (1984) Schmerz – Konzepte und ärztliches Handeln [Pain – concepts and medical approach]. Springer, Berlin

Index

A

Acute periarthritic pain attack, 92, 95, 96
Acute trauma, 71
Algodystrophie reflexe, 102
Algodystrophy, 107
Allodynia, 124
Alloparalgia, 125
Anamnesis, 68
Arteriography, of subclavian
    artery, 122–123
Axillary fascia, 103

B

Backlash injury, 36
Bicipital aponeurosis, 39, 53, 54
Bicipital fissure, radial nerve decompression
    in lateral, 75

C

Carpal tunnel syndrome, 84
Cauterisation, 1
Chronic trauma, 71
Complete temporary pain elimination
    technique, 95–97
Complex regional pain syndrome I (CRPS I)
    aetiology and pathogenesis, 108–111
    classification, 125
    complications, 127–128
    diagnostics, 111
        arteriography of subclavian artery,
            122–123
        brachial plexus and intraoperative
            findings, 124
        differential, 124–125
        phlebography of subclavian vein,
            117–122

tabular documentation of pathologic
    findings, 111–117
epidemiology, 106–107
examination sheet for patients with,
    112–113
indications and contraindications,
    125–126
mistakes, dangers and
    complications, 147
postoperative treatment, 134–136
preoperative findings, 114, 115
results, 138–143
surgically relevant anatomy and
    physiology, 102–106
surgical treatment
    history, 126–127
    informed patient consent, 127–128
    instruments, 128–129
    transaxillary decompression and
        resection of upper thoracic
        sympathetic trunk, 129–134
Coracoiditis, 123
Cubital fossa, 51–54

D

Deep radial branch, decompression of, 21
Distal compression mechanism, of ulnar
    nerve, 50
Dorsal horn synapsis system, pain inhibitory
    function of, 143–147
Double nerve lesion, 4

E

Epicondylitis. *see* Tennis Elbow (TE), 1
    and Golf Elbow (GE), 36

Epicondyle region
  lateral
    degenetation of, 21–27
    innervation of, 2–4
  medial
    denervation of, 48, 52
    innervation of, 34, 35
Epicondylitis lateralis humeri.
      See Tennis elbow (TE) 1–28
Epicondylopathy. *See* Tennis elbow (TE)
Epitrochleoanconaeus muscle, 40
  insertion and origin of, 41
ERCB, tendon, strain stress of, 7

F
Fascia, longitudinal incision of, 21
Fascial incision, lengthening of, 21
FCU. *See* Flexor carpi ulnaris
      muscle (FCU)
Fibrous arcade, resection of, 73–74
Flexor carpi ulnaris muscle
    (FCU), 36
  deep aponeurosis of, 49
Forearm positions, diverse effects of, 8
Frozen shoulder, 83

G
Golf elbow (GE)
  aetiology and pathogenesis, 36–37
  causes of, 38, 39
  classification, 46
  conservative treatment of, 46–47
  diagnostics, 44–45
  endogenous precondition for, 37
  epidemiology, 36
  indications and contraindications, 46
  mistakes, dangers and
      complications, 56
  neurogenous genesis of, 37–43
  neuro-irritation impulses, 38
  results, 54–55
  surgically relevant anatomy and
      physiology, 34–36
  surgical treatment
    anaesthesia and positioning, 47–49
    by denervation and decompression of
      ulnar nerve, 47–49
    of median nerve, 51–54
    and of median nerve, 47–54
    denervation and circumcision
      of medial epicondyle
      region, 47–49

    denervation and transposition of ulnar
      nerve, 49–51
    denervation and decompression of
      median nerve, 51–54
    informed patient consent, 47
    of resistant cases, 49–51

H
Hand-finger syndrome, 122
Hiatus scalenorum, 104

I
Irritation syndrome, of radial nerve, 4
Ischaemia test, 124

L
Ligamentary arcade, compressive
      effect of, 8–10
Luxation and subluxation, 49–51, of ulnar
      nerve, 51

M
Median compression, aetiology and
      pathogenesis of, 102–103
Memantine, 126, 146–147
Motbus Sudeck (RSD, CRPS I), 101
Multiple fasciotomies, 126
Myokinetic supinator syndrome, 69

N
Neuro-irritation impulses, 38
NMDA receptor, mechanism of, 147

P
Paget-von Schroetter syndrome, 84
Partial upper frontal shoulder quadrant
      denervation technique, 92–95
Periarthritic attack, 89
Phlebography, 91
  of subclavian vein, 117–122
Posttraumatic dystrophy, 101
Pronation and supination test of
      Werner (TE), 17
Proximal compression mechanism, 42
Proximal radial compression syndrome
    (PRKS)
  aetiology and pathogenesis, 63–68
  classification, 69–70

conservative treatment, 71
    indications for, 71
decompression of radial nerve,
        64–68, 72–75
    proximal of the lateral muscular
        ligament, 63, 64, 72–74
    (1st compression mechanism) resection of
        the radial nerve hiatus, 64, 75
    (2nd compression mechanism) resection of
        fibrous arcade distal of the radial
        nerve hiatus, 64, 73
    (3rd compression mechanism) decompres-
        sion in lateral bicipital fissure, 75
diagnostics, 68–69
epidemiology, 63
intraoperative findings, 74–75
mistakes, dangers and complications,
        78–80
results, 75–78
surgically relevant anatomy and
        physiology, 61–63
surgical treatment, 72
    anaesthesia and positioning, 72
    informed patient consent, 71–72
Proximal ulnar compression syndrome
        (PUKS), 36
Puncture, 95

R
Radial irritation syndrome (RIS), 62
Radial nerve
    decompression, 64–68, 72–74
    resection of hiatus ni. rods and fibrous
        arcade, 73
    in supinator-channel, 20
Radial styloiditis, 62
Raynaud's disease, 122
Reflectory trophoneurosis, 101
Reflex regional pain syndrome (CRPS I,
        Morbus Sudeck, RSD), 101
    aetiology and pathogenesis, 108–111
    classification, 125
    complications, 127–128
    diagnostics, 111
        arteriography of subclavian artery,
            122–123
        brachial plexus and intraoperative
            findings, 124
        differential, 124–125
        phlebography of subclavian vein,
            117–122
        tabular documentation of pathologic
            findings, 111–117

epidemiology, 106–107
indications and contraindications,
        125–126
mistakes, dangers and complications, 147
postoperative treatment, 134–136
preoperative findings, 114, 115
results, 138–143
surgically relevant anatomy and
        physiology, 102–106
surgical treatment
    history, 126–127
    informed patient consent, 127–128
    instruments, 128–129
    transaxillary decompression,
            129–134
RIS. See Radial irritation syndrome (RIS)
RSD. See Reflex sympathetic
        dystrophy (RSD)

S
Scalene muscle, 104, 105
Scalenopleural muscle, 104
SD. See Sudeck's dystrophy (SD)
Shoulder joint pain syndrome
    classification, 92
    diagnostics, 89–92
    epidemiology, 88
    etiology and pathogenesis, 88–89
    indications and contraindications, 92
    mistakes, dangers and complications, 98
    results, 97–98
    surgically relevant anatomy and
            physiology, 84–87
    therapy
        complete temporary pain elimination
                technique, 95–97
        partial upper frontal shoulder
                quadrant denervation technique,
                92–95
Sibson fascia, 105
Skin incision, 20–26
Subclavian artery
    arteriography of, 122–123
    pathologic findings at, 122
Subclavian vein, phlebography of, 117–122
Sudeck's dystrophy (SD), 96, 102, 111
    diagnosis of, 114
    pathogenesis of, 110
    phlebographic findings in, 117–119
    symptoms of, 115
Superior thoracic vessels, 103
Supinator arcade, intraoperative presentation of, 7
Supinator syndrome, 69

T

TE. *See* Tennis elbow (TE)

Tendinogenous pathogenesis, promoters of, 37

Tendinous origin, radial nerve
    decompression in, 72–73

Tennis elbow (TE), 1
    aetiology and pathogenesis of, 5–16
    classification, 17
    conservative treatment of, 18–19
    decompression of radial nerve, 19
    diagnostics, 16–17
    epidemiology, 5
    incidence of, 5
    indications and contraindications, 17–18
    mistakes, dangers and complications,
        28–29
    postoperative treatment, 27
    results, 27–28
    surgically relevant anatomy and
        physiology, 2–5
    surgical treatment
        anaesthesia and positioning, 20
        informed patient consent, 19–20
        skin incision, 20–26
    symptoms of, 16

Thoracic inlet syndrome (TIS), 69

Thoracic outlet, 103

Thoracic outlet syndrome (TOS), 88, 90, 96
    examination sheet for patients
        with, 112–113
    treatment of, 102

Thrower elbow. *See* Golf elbow (GE)

TIS. *See* Thoracic inlet syndrome
    (TIS)

TOS. *See* Thoracic outlet syndrome
    (TOS)

Transaxillary decompression, surgical
    technique of, 129–134

Triceps muscle, overexertion of, 71

U

Ulnar nerve
    distal compression mechanism
        of, 50
    irritation, 36
    luxation of, 40, 50, 51
    subluxation of, 40, 48

Upper arm, radial nerve decompression
    in, 76

Upper extremity
    partial radial paresis of, 75, 77
    pathologic findings at, 111–117

V

Venous stasis, 116

Venous stenosis, 106

W

Wartenberg syndrome, 69